302

UNIVERSITY OF OXFORD
CENTRE FOR SOCIO-LEGAL
STUDIES

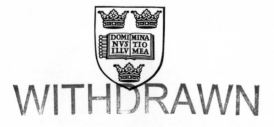

THE PATRICK AND CAROLINE
NEILL LIBRARY

NO FEET TO DRAG

No Feet to Drag
Report on the DISABLED

ALFRED MORRIS

and ARTHUR BUTLER

SIDGWICK & JACKSON
LONDON

First published in Great Britain

Copyright © 1972 by Alfred Morris and Arthur Butler

I.S.B.N. 0.283.97867. 8

Printed in Great Britain by
Eden Fisher (Southend) Ltd
for Sidgwick and Jackson Limited
1 Tavistock Chambers, Bloomsbury Way
London W.C.1A 2SG

Contents

~~~~~~

List of Illustrations

~~~~~~~~~~~~~~~~~~~~~~~~~~~~~~~~~

Acknowledgements

The photographs are reproduced with the kind permission of *The Sunday People*, the Press Association, the Disabled Drivers' Association, the *Hornsey Journal*, and the Spastics Society

Prologue

~~~~~~~~~~~~~~~~~~~~~~~~~~~~~~~~~~~~~

by Alfred Morris

My father died as one of the tubercular poor before I was eight years old. He was forty-four at his death on 11 November 1935. There was a strange irony in the date. It was a sharp reminder that *heart failure, accelerated by tuberculosis* (in the words of the death certificate) was much more the occasion than the cause of my father's death. For he was a disabled ex-serviceman of the savage and mindless war which had ended seventeen years to the day before he died. He had multiple handicaps, from severe leg injuries to partial blindness, and in recent years had become chronically sick from the deficiency disease that hastened his death. In 1918-19, Manchester was a hospital city with thirty thousand beds for the war wounded. As a patient there at Grangethorpe Hospital, my father was in the care of Professor (now Sir) Harry Platt, the distinguished ortho-paedic surgeon who fifty years later, as President of the Central Council for the Disabled, was to work with me as a close colleague in the making of the Chronically Sick and Disabled Persons Act 1970.

My father was a sign-writer by trade, but only rarely by occupation. Towards the end of his life it was usually impossible for him to find employment, even for the short periods when he was well enough to go to work. With mass unemployment among the able-bodied, it is not surprising that there were few employment opportunities for the chronically sick and disabled. When he died, in

Withington Hospital, Manchester, a public official pointedly suggested to my mother that, instead of her arranging the funeral from home with a private undertaker, my father could be taken for burial from the hospital to nearby Southern Cemetery direct, in order to save unnecessary expense. This was deeply insensitive and wounding to my mother. We were then unavoidably in receipt of public assistance, but notwithstanding all her customary kindliness and fortitude my mother, who survived my father by twenty-four years of widowhood, could never forget the cruel insult that had been added to her bereavement. My father was buried from home, but in a grave without a stone. In the 1930s, even more than in the post-war years, disablement was another word for poverty. My mother would have said that it was often also another word for needless humiliation.

When she sought to confirm her right to a war-widow's pension, my mother found officialdom as intractable as it had previously been insensitive. I think we were first told that my father's war pension had died with him, or words to that effect, on the grounds that his death was not directly due to the injuries for which his pension had been awarded. The battle to reverse this decision was dour and protracted. The late Alderman Harry Thorneycroft, our Member of Parliament, was eventually asked to intervene on my mother's behalf. It was only then, some years after my father's death, that my mother's status as a war widow was confirmed. The battle raged long enough to leave me with a lasting interest in war pensions and the war disabled. From Harry Thorneycroft, who later became a personal friend, I learned what may well be the golden rule for any public representative. He always at least tried to put the same valuation on a letter as the constituent who wrote to him. He saw that few people write to their Members of Parliament simply for the sake of writing. He knew also that just one letter out of a hundred in his weekly postbag could be the only letter written in that year by a constituent in need. As well as being a man of marked generosity and understanding, Harry Thorneycroft was more than a match for the more pompous ornaments of officialdom. He and my mother would have been happy to know that I was subsequently to introduce legislation to amend the War Pensions Act 1921 and the Pensions Appeal Tribunals Act 1943, both to speed and simplify pension procedures for disabled ex-servicemen.

My parents spent most of their short married life as the tenants of 34, Gray Street, an aged, crumbling and long since demolished terraced slum in the Ancoats district of Manchester. It was one of the most deprived localities in the city and ours was among the poorest homes in Ancoats. Mancunians have long taken pride in preserving some of the quaint fourteenth-century buildings in the Old Shambles area of the city, near to Manchester Cathedral. Ancoats was our New Shambles, which almost everyone living there wanted to tear down. There was nothing quaint or endearing about the architecture of Ancoats. Thrown up by speculative builders in the nineteenth century, its mostly verminous homes were as ugly as their structures were unsound. In Alfred Lord Tennyson's phrase: ... *there rain'd a ghastly dew*.

Nor were the schools any prettier than the jerry-built houses. The very term 'educational priority area' must have been invented by someone who lived in unreconstructed Ancoats. But at least for my brothers and sisters, as well as for me, school was warmer and drier than home. Ours was a house that 'rained in' more than most in the neighbourhood and it was all hands on the upper deck when the rains came. Catching the raindrops in a bucket was a bedroom skill at which even the pre-school child had to excel in the Ancoats of my childhood. We never compared our condition with that of children elsewhere, because most of us seldom, if ever, moved out of our immediate neighbourhood. While I lived in Ancoats it is unlikely that I ever moved more than a mile away from Gray Street. There was simply no occasion to go beyond the undifferentiated streets of Ancoats, least of all for children whose fathers were disabled.

Shortly before my father's death, we moved from the slums as beneficiaries of a modest but imaginative scheme promoted by Canon Shimwell, of All Souls Church, Ancoats,

for the re-housing of very poor families. My father's unemployment, not to say unemployability by that time, left
my parents unlikely to qualify for a council house as they
could not have guaranteed regular payment of the rent.
In those days, council houses in Manchester mostly went to
working people who were in secure employment, such as
railwaymen, postmen, bus and tram drivers and conductors.
This meant that many of the poorest families, however
badly they were housed, had little hope of being re-housed
on the city's new housing estates. Under Canon Shimwell's
scheme, which was financed by individual loans at nominal
rates of interest, we were re-housed in a house very much like
a council house in Newton Heath, Manchester. The original
rent was 11s. 3d. per week, compared with 10s. 0d. for 34,
Gray Street. In Newton Heath, we had not only a weather-
proof home, a bath and other modern conveniences, but
even a small garden. For my father, however, the move
had come much too late. He was now unable to stray very
far from the living room of our new home. Indeed, my
memory is of him sitting immovable in a chair, as if defeated
even by the weight of the blanket round his shoulders.
Even as we arrived in Newton Heath, there was not the
merest chance that he would ever enjoy the benefits of his
merciful release from the squalor and decay of Gray Street.
He was fatally ill.

Although still less than eight years old, I had already
experienced the realities of life for a disabled family. Ever
since my childhood I have known that the quickest way
to find a deprived child is first to find a disabled father.
Even if the disabled father is employed, he will usually be
working in menial and, therefore, low-paid employment.
If he is unemployed, in most cases he and his family will be
living at or near subsistence level. By definition of the word
family, if one member is disabled, then the family as a whole
is disabled. The child of a severely disabled parent is just
as much involved in the problems of severe disablement
as the parent of a disabled child. Whenever a severely
disabled person is handicapped socially, for example, by
avoidable restrictions on his mobility or his exclusion from

inaccessible public and social buildings, his family also is socially handicapped. There are things other families can do that they cannot do. There are places other families can visit that they cannot visit. That is why I emphasized, throughout the parliamentary debates on my Bill, the deep importance of the concept of the disabled family. It is also why I have stated as a fact that, in contemporary Britain, there are many millions of people who are personally involved in the problems of severe disablement who are not themselves disabled.

When I was married in September 1950, after service in the army and before entering the University of Oxford, I went to live at the home of my wife's parents in the very poor Collyhurst district of Manchester. I had left school and started work at fourteen, but had continued my education at evening schools in Manchester until entering the army at eighteen. My wife's parents lived at 10, Laverack Street, Collyhurst, which, like 34, Gray Street in the 1930s, was aching for demolition. It was another two-up-and-two-down gas-lit slum terrace, with one cold-water tap and an old iron stove in a tiny scullery off the back yard, a penny-in-the-slot gas meter for cooking and lighting, an outside lavatory and a prodigiously-leaking roof. We were constantly doing minor repairs, but whenever the question of major repairs was raised with the landlord he always reacted as if we were joking. In justification of his reaction, I think it should be said that it would have been more hazardous and costly to repair than to rebuild.

My wife's mother was totally incapacitated by rheumatoid arthritis and could move about only if pushed in her wheelchair. She was a deeply religious woman, but it was a daunting struggle for her even to attend the Anglican church some eighty yards from her home. My wife's father, Abel Jones, a wagon sheet repairer on the railways until his final illness in 1951, was a victim of chronic bronchitis and ultimately of dropsy. His bronchitis originated in severe gassing while serving with the Manchester Regiment in the First World War, in which he became a prisoner-of-war at the age of eighteen. Even while my father-in-law was awaiting admission to Crumpsall Hospital, where he died, his bed, which was then on the ground floor in the living room of the house, was sometimes dampened by rain from the leaking roof. As well as being one of the most intelligent men I have known, he was also one of the most calm, gentle and considerate. He knew that he would never return home from Crumpsall Hospital, but was much more concerned for his wife than for himself.

By then, although my wife still worked in Manchester and looked after her parents, Laverack Street was my home for only twenty-eight weeks of the year. For the other twenty-four weeks I was in Oxford in the Honours School of Modern History. With one foot in Oxford and the other in Collyhurst, and having travelled widely at home and abroad in the army, I was now well able to contrast widely differing standards of domestic comfort. In Oxford, I lived at the home of the late Philip Andrews, a Fellow both of New College and Nuffield. He was a staunch Conservative with a passionate belief in the theory of economic rent. But his precepts were not his practice. He was much too kindly a man to charge me anything like the economic rent of the spacious accommodation he provided. There is no need to dwell here on the preventable suffering inflicted on my wife's mother by her environment. Merely to describe the housing conditions in which she, and countless others like her, had to live is to indict public authority for its utter neglect of the housing needs of severely disabled people. As the law then stood, and was to remain until it was altered by the Chronically Sick and Disabled Persons Act 1970, there was no requirement whatever upon local housing authorities to make special provision for the housing needs of the disabled.

Two years after my wife's father died, we were offered a council flat in Wythenshawe. This was not because my wife's mother was severely disabled. It was simply that we had finally reached the top of Manchester's housing waiting list. The flat we moved into was on the southernmost edge of the city and backed on to open fields in the Cheshire countryside. For my mother-in-law and my wife, it was their first experience of living in a home with electricity, inside plumbing and a fixed bath. Even here, however, there were intimidating problems for the disabled family. Baths can become a mockery for those who cannot use them. In the case of my wife's mother, it was necessary for her to be lifted in and out of the bath. She suffered many indignities which a hoist could have prevented. Ramps, handrails, a raised lavatory seat and other housing adaptations would also have added to the comfort and dignity of her final years. We had no private transport and my mother-in-law's world was limited to the distance her wheelchair could be pushed by my wife and by me. We attempted to go on a family holiday once, but only once. For my wife's mother it was not so much a holiday, more a test of endurance. There were very few social buildings she could ever hope to enter and even churchgoing was now too difficult to attempt. This was especially sad. In effect, it was the breaking of her final link with any social group beyond the home. But she never complained. She talked more of the crippled people who were left in the damp and dirt of Collyhurst, including former neighbours who lived alone, than of her own deprivations in our healthier new environment. As the contemporary poet, Tony Connor, would have put it for her:

> *My mind runs on, and back, and round,*
> *. . . I cannot now escape*
> *Shadowy entries, streets that wind,*
> *alleys that are often blind.*

This was some of the personal background that informed my desire to make life better, and safer, for the chronically sick and disabled and their families when I became the Member of Parliament for Wythenshawe in October, 1964. My early public life, before entering the House of Commons, had brought me into contact with many families like my own, in Liverpool as well as Manchester.* I learned more of the problems of chronically sick young people in long-stay

---

*At the age of twenty-three, Alfred Morris was the Labour candidate for the Garston division of Liverpool at the General Election of October 1951. He became prospective Labour candidate for Manchester, Wythenshawe, in December, 1955, gaining the seat in 1964.

hospital accommodation, of the special educational difficulties of handicapped children and of the anguish of elderly disabled people struggling, often against hopeless odds, to preserve their independence. I knew that very few such people wanted to become institutionalized if they could possibly remain independent. I knew also that the cost to public funds of hospital and other institutional care is almost always higher than the cost of aiding them to live in the community, with adequate help and facilities in the home. Then there were the problems of the disabled housewife. There were cases known to me of disabled housewives being splashed in the face by hot fat while making meals for their families, simply because no one had ever thought of designing a gas or electric cooker adjusted to the working height of women in wheelchairs.

I became involved also in helping mentally handicapped people to rejoin the community. In one case, I secured the release of a Manchester man, Jim Johnson, who had been held for twenty-odd years in the mental hospital at Calderstones, near Blackburn. As a child, he had suffered injuries in a road accident, which kept him away from school and led to his becoming educationally sub-normal. He had been put in grim Calderstones as an adolescent, after a petty theft from a gas meter for which he was held responsible. On his release, he was found work as a Manchester dustman and his only eccentricity was to report for work half an hour before he was due. He has now lived with his disabled sister in Wythenshawe, and has been a taxpayer, since 1960 without any question of his being returned to a mental institution. His sister never believed that Jim had committed the theft. She had made the long return journey to visit her brother in Calderstones every week while he was there. Other problems in which I became involved were those of disablement income and of working men whose severely disabled wives had to be left alone in their homes throughout the working day. I was aware of the invaluable work done by the Manchester and Salford Cripples' Help Society, the Manchester and Salford Blind Aid Society and their many sister organizations. Without their voluntary help, the lives of many thousands of severely disabled people would have been even more wretched. I knew as well that the local authorities with which I was familiar were among the more concerned to use their existing powers in the welfare field. But clearly, their powers were totally inadequate to deal with a challenge on the scale then facing public authority.

While I was at the University of Oxford, one of the required texts for my special subject in the Honours School of Modern History was *Conditions of the Working Class in England in 1844*, by Friedrich Engels. I had not been a Member of Parliament long before feeling it was time someone wrote a parallel book on the conditions of the chronically sick and disabled in Britain in the second half of the twentieth century. Engels had shocked many of his Victorian contemporaries by describing the blighted lives and environment, the privations and avoidable suffering, of the industrial poor in mid-nineteenth-century England. What seemed to be needed now was a text that would arouse feeling for the very large numbers of people in contemporary Britain who were mostly never seen in society. In far too many cases, they were never seen simply because they were locked away, not just in institutions but in so-called homes, houses and flats alike, that were not built for the needs of severely handicapped people and served only as prisons without trial. But it was a time for action more than for essays. There were more and more people outside, as well as within the two Houses of Parliament, who were now determined to change and humanize the law. Metaphorically speaking, the disabled were on the march and we were marching with them.

When I won the opportunity to legislate in the Private Members' Ballot of November, 1969, there was no expensively pre-packed Bill for me to present to the House of Commons. It has been said that my only possessions were a blank piece of paper and a burning conviction. But there was never any doubt what problems I would tackle. When the title of my Bill was announced, I was frequently asked what kind of improvements for the chronically sick and disabled I had in mind. It always seemed best to begin with the problems of access. I explained that I wanted to remove the severe and gratuitous social handicaps inflicted on disabled people, and often on their families and friends, not just by their exclusion from town and county halls, art galleries, libraries and many of the universities, but even from pubs, restaurants, theatres, cinemas and other places of entertainment. Steps without ramps, no less than sharp, twisting staircases, narrow corridors and awkward doorways, can bar a person in a wheelchair, or using walking aids, as effectively as locked and bolted doors. With parliamentary colleagues who worked with me on my Bill, I knew that opening doors to the disabled was of fundamental importance to improving their social status. Their forced exclusion from public and social buildings makes them feel like a race apart. In seeking to throw open the doors of these buildings, I explained that I and my friends were concerned to stop society from treating disabled people as if they were a separate species.

Among the most sensitive problems we announced that we would tackle were those of the young chronic sick languishing in geriatric wards, and of the young and homeless disabled living among mostly very elderly residents in local authority welfare homes. In consultation with Marsh Dickson, of the National Campaign for the Young Chronic Sick, a man of wide experience in this field, I had asked numerous parliamentary questions about these problems. Yet I had been unable even to discover how many young people were so confined. We knew that we could not hope to add years to the lives of these young people, but at least we could try to add life to their years. Then there were the problems of housing for severely disabled people living at home, the special educational problems of severely handicapped children, mobility and employment problems and many others, including the need to make sure that the disabled were given their proper place in advising Ministers and other policy-makers on decisions affecting their lives. There was also the need to increase spending on technological aids and research and development in the service of

disabled people. For military purposes, resources for research and development were plentiful. But for the purpose
of helping to normalize the lives of the disabled, such
resources were extremely scarce.

There were two other compelling and related needs.
First, to obtain full identification of the severely disabled
in Britain. Without this, policy-making is blind. And second,
to provide a high general standard of local authority services
that would enable severely disabled people to live in decency
and dignity in their own homes. Most of all, we were determined to ensure, by changing the law, that it would no
longer be possible for anyone in public authority to say that
he did not know the full size of the disablement problem.
In 1969 there were only 235,000 on the disablement registers
kept by local authorities. But there was clear evidence
that the real figure was at least one and a half million.
This meant that there were perhaps upwards of one million
severely disabled men, women and children in need of help
whose identities were unknown to public authority.

This was the most sombre of our reflections when we
began to draft my Chronically Sick and Disabled Persons
Bill. Even the keeping of local disablement registers was
permissive. The local councils could virtually decide for
themselves whether such registers should be kept. They were
kept under Section 29 of the National Assistance Act 1948,
and recorded the cases only of people receiving some kind
of help from the council. They were certainly *not* registers
of the actual incidence of severe disablement in any locality.
In Kingston-upon-Hull, 10·8 per thousand of the local
population were registered as disabled, while in Solihull
the figure was only 0·9 per thousand. This made it appear
that the incidence of severe disablement in Kingston-upon-
Hull was twelve times as high as in Solihull. In fact, however, such sharp apparent differences had more to do with
whether local services were good or bad (or almost non-
existent) than with any real difference in the numbers of
people who were severely disabled. Local authority services
for the disabled were as permissive as registration and they
too were based on Section 29 of the 1948 Act. We knew it

would be essential to amend that Act if we were to ensure a high general standard of local services. Knowing also how little most local authorities were then providing, we were determined to disturb their smug complacency and make them do for the chronically sick and disabled what they had failed to do when given the option.

What follows in this book is a deeply disturbing picture by my friend, Arthur Butler, of the sadly intimidating problems that faced Britain's severely handicapped people and their families as my Bill was transformed into the Chronically Sick and Disabled Persons Act 1970. The difficulties of legislating, as a Private Member, about the duties of so many departments of state, of hospital and other public boards and of every major local authority, are also discussed. There is full acknowledgement of the very substantial progress made by the many and diverse public authorities which have begun to make the Act a meaningful reality. This is not allowed to cloak the dilatoriness of other public authorities which could have moved with much greater speed and humanity. It is shown in the pages that follow that both the voluntary organizations and the media have been determined to spotlight the tragic human cost of lethargy by any public authority. The voluntary organizations waited far too long for comprehensive legislation on disablement to let it go by default in any locality. This too is fully recognized in the pages that follow. I have attempted, in the final chapter, to point the way towards further improvement in social provision for the chronically sick and disabled. The new goals will not be easy to achieve, but it is a prerequisite of further improvement rapidly to increase public awareness of the appalling conditions in which even many of the most severely handicapped people have had to exist in contemporary Britain. For further improvement it is also perhaps essential to realize that, potentially, we are *all* disabled.

~~~~~~

Chapter One

The Missing Million

BRITAIN'S POLITICIANS – with a few notable exceptions in both main parties – have no cause to be proud of their record on behalf of the disabled. For years, indeed up to the Alfred Morris Bill and the tremendous publicity that surrounded it, M.P.s seemed strangely unaware of the acute and special problems of what amounted to a very considerable proportion of the population. To take the most cynical view, as a parliamentary journalist must sometimes be excused for doing, the fact that leading politicians had no idea that so many people were suffering from disablement, and that so many votes were involved, probably had something to do with the neglect of the subject at Westminster.

Within the Labour Movement only the Co-operative Party, the smallest but often the most radical and socially alert of its three wings, had devoted much attention to the problems of this, the most hard-pressed section of the community. The Co-operative Party had passed resolutions year after year at its annual conference on the need to provide better care for the aged, including the disabled. One of the first speeches made by Alfred Morris at a Co-operative conference was in a debate on this issue long before he entered Parliament. There is something about the tradition of good neighbourliness in the Co-operative movement that makes its members particularly sensitive to welfare problems in the community. Generally speaking it chooses to be represented in Parliament by men and women who are deeply concerned to do something practical to help the needy.

It was as a Labour and Co-operative member that Alfred Morris entered Parliament in 1964. He had been sent there by the voters of Wythenshawe in the General Election that put Labour in power with a wafer-thin majority that was to fluctuate between five and one for the next seventeen months. There had been no mention of the problems of the disabled in the election manifestos either of the Labour Party or the defeated Tories. Moreover, there had been no debate in the House of Commons on the subject since the previous General Election of 1959. As a political issue it was non-existent.

One reason for this lack of interest stemmed from the fact that the disabled are not a homogeneous group speaking with one voice through some central organization. It has become common practice to talk of the disabled, and sometimes to treat them, as though they are a separate and distinct race of people. But disabled people are as various as those who have not yet suffered the misfortune of disablement. Groups of people suffering from the same disabilities had organized themselves, and various voluntary agencies had been set up to work on behalf of some sections of the disabled population. The blind and war disabled were two of the first groups to receive such assistance. But hundreds of thousands of disabled people were spread throughout Britain, unrecognized, unregistered and unaided by the authorities.

They had medical problems and housing problems; problems of education and training; of employment and income; of mobility and access; of leisure and equipment. But a large number had no desire to be organized or registered just for the sake of being registered. This was to be recognized later by Alfred Morris who stressed in Parliament the importance of confidentiality and voluntaryism to most disabled people. They had no wish to be labelled as special cases or to go cap-in-hand seeking charity. They just wanted to live as much as possible like completely able-bodied people – to live as normally as possible in their own homes, amongst their own families. The great majority also had a very real desire to do their bit for the family and the community through a job of work.

Disparate and diverse, the disabled had come to be treated by the Government in a piecemeal and haphazard fashion. A large number of different Whitehall departments had become involved over the years in dealing with a number of their problems, such as medical services, welfare, education, training and employment. This unco-ordinated Whitehall approach, with each department jealously guarding its own little sector of the front, had led a number of committees of inquiry to criticize the system. But their reports, like so many others, were gathering dust on Whitehall shelves. What no one appears to have seen is that, since responsibility for the disabled was scattered all across Whitehall, only an informed back bench M.P., with no departmental jealousies, was likely ever to suggest comprehensive legislation.

The legislation which formed the basis of the Whitehall effort had been inspired by both humanitarian and utilitarian considerations. The legislators had been anxious not only to give a helping hand to certain types of disabled people, but also to ensure that any capable of working were helped to do so in the interest of economy. It took the carnage of two world wars to spur the politicians into fitful action. The first legislation specifically for the disabled was the Blind Persons Act of 1920. The Government also set up instructional factories for disabled ex-servicemen – one of whom was Alfred Morris's father. The State moved into action again during the Second World War with the Disabled Persons Employment Act, 1944. It was presented to Parliament as a first attempt to treat the subjects of rehabilitation and resettlement as a single problem. The aim was to get the medical and industrial worlds to co-operate in the interests of the handicapped. It was followed up by another Act in 1958, but the only war preceding that piece of legislation was the Suez fiasco in which the main casualties were Britain's pride and reputation as a Great Power.

For the next ten years Whitehall was content to administer

these Acts and no major initiatives were forthcoming from Governments. In fact, the credit for progress made in legislation in recent years must go to a handful of dedicated back-benchers on both sides of the Commons – and Lords. But not even these Parliamentary campaigners would have accomplished what they have without the work of the voluntary agencies and such forceful and inspiring crusaders as the late Megan du Boisson, founder of the Disablement Income Group, Marsh Dickson of the National Campaign for the Young Chronic Sick, Duncan Guthrie, director of the Central Council for the Disabled, James Loring, director of the Spastics Society, Lady Hamilton of the Disabled Living Foundation, Donald Powell of the British Polio Fellowship; A. C. Waine, General Secretary of the Multiple Sclerosis Society, Ian Henderson, General Secretary of the British Council for Rehabilitation of the Disabled, and many others.

It is, therefore, a pity that since the passing of the Morris Act a few politicians have sought to make party political capital out of the fact that this Private Member's Bill – which won the support of all parties – reached the Statute Book in the lifetime of a Labour Government. It can be shown, in fact, that at the outset the member of Mr Wilson's Cabinet most concerned with the problems of the disabled was distinctly lukewarm in his reaction to the Bill. Moreover, from ministers' speeches during the passage of the Bill, it is questionable whether Labour, if it had been returned to office in 1970, would have quickly gone all out to get a 100 per cent register compiled of Britain's disabled. Much would have depended on who became minister.

It was following Labour's return to power in 1966 that back-bench pressure began to build up for a better deal for the disabled. Meanwhile, behind the scenes in Whitehall the department most concerned was absorbed in preparing a massive National Superannuation and Social Insurance Bill. 'The half-pay on retirement' Bill as it had become known to the press and public was aimed to replace flat-rate by earnings-related contributions, and the minister responsible for its preparation was Richard Crossman, Secretary of State for Health and Social Security, a political innovator of high intelligence. Linked with this highly complicated measure were some proposals that had an important bearing on the financial problems of the disabled. There was to be a constant attendance allowance of £4 a week for those so severely disabled (including disabled wives and the parents of badly handicapped children) that they required constant attendance from another person. The Labour Government estimated that some 50,000 people would qualify. There was also to be a new earnings-related benefit known as an invalidity pension which would be payable after twenty-eight weeks of illness.

But there had been no reference to the problems of the disabled in Labour's 1966 election manifesto – and only a passing reference to severe disability in the Tory manifesto.

On the back-benches, however, both Conservative and Labour M.P.s had attempted to deal with various problems of the disabled in Private Members' Bills in the few years before Alfred Morris introduced his measure. One of the most memorable attempts was made in July 1968 by Jack Ashley, Labour M.P. for Stoke-on-Trent South. Ashley, a one-time labourer, crane driver and shop steward, had won a scholarship to Ruskin College, Oxford, and from there had gone to Cambridge where he became President of the Union. After working as a B.B.C. Television producer he had entered the Commons in 1966 and appeared all set for a brilliant parliamentary career when he was struck by total deafness. At first he decided to give up his Commons seat but he was persuaded by friends to stay on. He did a crash course in lip-reading – helped by his wife, Pauline. She was in the gallery when he sought permission of the House to bring in a Bill to set up a Commission to investigate the problems of the disabled and tackle anomalies in their treatment.

Ashley pointed out that a husband totally disabled with multiple sclerosis received only one third as much as a man suffering from an industrial injury. He argued that even Iceland made better provision for its disabled men and women. There were about 200 M.P.s in the House to hear his speech. He could not hear their cheers at the end but he could see from their reaction that he had succeeded in his attempt to introduce the Bill. Unfortunately, it was very near the end of that session of Parliament. The exercise was unable to achieve more than publicity for the cause.

In November 1968 a Conservative back-bencher introduced a Bill to tackle another aspect of the problem. He was James Prior, member for Lowestoft, a Suffolk farmer who had been educated at Charterhouse and Cambridge. Prior was also Parliamentary Private Secretary to the Leader of the Opposition, Mr Edward Heath. He had won fifth place in the annual ballot among back-benchers to introduce Private Members' Bills. The first dozen in the draw stand a chance of getting enough Commons time to push through a Bill. Prior, well-placed at number five, chose to help housewives and others not covered by National Insurance, industrial injuries or war disability schemes, who had been handicapped by such illnesses as muscular dystrophy, multiple sclerosis, arthritis, thrombosis and polio. He also sought to give ministers powers to direct local authorities to reserve a proportion of council houses for the disabled and equip them with special fitments. It was estimated that about 200,000 disabled housewives and 140,000 men and women disabled since childhood would qualify for the first time for a pension under his Bill. In February, however, the Bill was rejected by the Commons by 112 to 76 votes. An angry Tory M.P. described the Labour Government's forces which had voted down the measure as 'the payroll vote plus two volunteers'.

Meanwhile, in December 1968 another Tory back-bencher, Mr Gordon Campbell (Moray and Nairn) backed by M.P.s of all parties, published a Bill proposing an advisory commission to review pensions and benefits for the disabled. It was similar to the one introduced by Jack Ashley the previous July, but included some changes designed to make it more acceptable to the Government. Nevertheless, it was rejected in March by a derisory Commons vote of 28 to 24.

The annual ballot for Private Members' Bills came round again in November 1969. Alfred Morris, on a Parliamentary delegation to India, was unable to enter himself. But he had arranged for his brother Charles, M.P. for Manchester,

Openshaw, and the Government's deputy chief whip, to step into the breach. He entered his brother's name. The result of the ballot was announced on 6 November. Flying back to London from New Delhi two days later Alfred Morris picked up a day-old copy of *The Guardian*. He read that he had won first place.

By the time he arrived home he found a sackful of suggested subjects plus many draft Bills awaiting him. They had been sent to him by all kinds of organizations and pressure groups. Any M.P. in such a position must be very tempted to choose for his subject a Bill already drafted by some worthy body. The Government also has pet Bills suitable for Private Members' legislation. The late Arthur Skeffington, then Parliamentary Secretary to the Ministry of Housing and Local Government, had such a Bill which he sent to Morris. It dealt with the preservation of trees and it was ultimately taken up by Duncan Sandys, the former Tory Defence Minister who had won a lower place in the ballot.

But Morris had a pet subject of his own. Since he had entered the Commons in 1964 he had tabled many questions to ministers about the problems of the disabled. A lot of the answers had been far from satisfactory. He had seen the hardship and distress caused by disability in his own family. Now he had the opportunity to tackle some of the causes of this hardship. But among the impressive pile of suggestions and draft Bills sent to him there was none on disablement. He consulted his friends at Westminster. Some suggested that although it was a worthy and humane subject, it was not one that would excite the interest of the press and public and would not, therefore, make headline news. How wrong they were. Morris in any case was not interested in capturing the headlines. Others encouraged him to go ahead with a Bill on disablement. One such friend was Fred Peart, then holding the influential post of Lord President of the Council and Leader of the Commons. Morris was Parliamentary Private Secretary to Peart and they shared identical views about Britain joining the Common Market. They were also among the closest personal friends in the Commons. Three years

earlier Morris had been on a list of Parliamentary Private
Secretaries to be sacked for failing to vote with the Government on a three-line Whip in the Commons vote to enter
negotiations with Europe. The list had been issued by Harold
Wilson but Peart, then Minister of Agriculture, who had
appointed Morris as his Parliamentary Private Secretary
on the day he entered Parliament in 1964, had virtually
ignored the order from Downing Street and Morris continued to operate as his unpaid parliamentary aide. (He
was later officially re-instated by the Prime Minister.)

On Peart's suggestion Morris went to see Richard
Crossman, the member of the Cabinet most intimately
concerned with the problems of the disabled as Secretary
of State for Health and Social Security. Crossman had done
much in his career to identify areas of need in the welfare
state and to sort out priorities. He asked to see the draft
Bill. When Morris confessed that he had not yet prepared
one the minister asked instead if he had ever thought of
introducing a Bill on organ transplants. There was a suggestion of some drafting assistance if he would consider
a Bill on this alternative subject. This was a poor start
and few would have seen much prospect of getting anything
done. Perhaps it was because he was so busy launching his
mammoth Bill to bring in the ambitious new graduated
State Pension Scheme that Crossman appeared not to
appreciate the possibilities of a wide-ranging measure to aid
the chronically sick and disabled and their families.

Whatever the reason, even to senior colleagues Crossman's
attitude appeared to be that if he had thought that action was
necessary and urgent he would have introduced legislation
himself. But, as was soon to be shown, a comprehensive
measure to help the disabled involved many Whitehall
departments and only someone in a position to take more
than a solitary departmental view of the problem could see
the scope and potential of such a measure. Alfred Morris
reported back to his friends on Crossman's counter-sugges-
tion. They were disappointed but encouraged him to continue with his plan. He had only a blank sheet of paper and
a fortnight left of the twenty days in which, under Commons

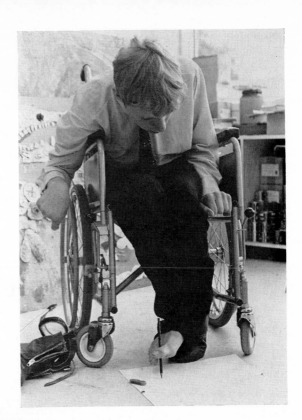

adly handicapped pupil at
Spastics Society's Thomas
rue School, Tonbridge, Kent,
ning to write with his foot.

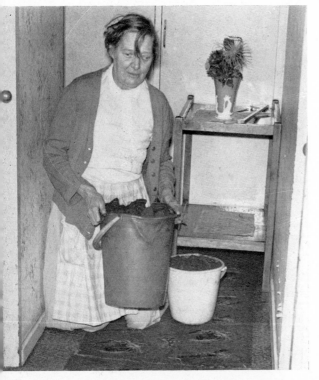

Mrs Dorothy Fisher, who has one leg amputated below the knee, was fifty-three when this picture was taken of her dragging coal from the bunker outside the front door to the room that served as living-room and bedroom for herself and her crippled husband.

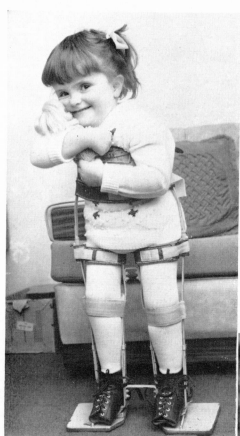

Sharon Neild was four years and five months old when this picture was taken. In that short time the little girl had already been through six major operations and five minor ones. Each time she has had an operation her doll Lulu has been taken to hospital to have one, too.

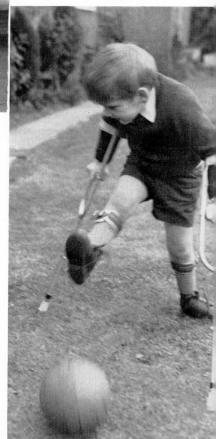

Jamie, a victim since birth of spina bifida, gets around with both legs in calipers and a pair of mini crutches. Aged five in January 1972 he is as ready as any other youngster for a game of football.

rules, he must produce the long title of the Bill. He then had another week before he had to produce the Bill itself. He quickly discovered that part of the advantage of winning first place in the ballot was lost by the fact that the winner had less time than any of the others in which to produce his measure. Some three weeks is a desperately short time in which to start from scratch to write a brand new Parliamentary Bill of major social importance.

One of the first moves that had to be made to start filling up the blank sheets was to encourage any Whitehall departments with ideas in their pending trays to hand them over.

Fred Peart offered to have Whitehall trawled for ideas, but the trawl produced only one immediate catch. Fred Mulley, then Minister of Transport, came up with a proposal to help thalidomide children and other disabled people by letting them use their powered wheelchairs on the pavements. The first reaction of the Department of the Environment, incorporating the Ministry of Housing, was not encouraging but later on this ministry, like many others, including Crossman's, was to become very helpful. Meanwhile, voluntary organizations concerned with the chronically sick and disabled were coming forward with their pet projects, and so were back-bench M.P.s who had taken an interest in various aspects of the problem. On the Labour side these M.P.s included Jack Ashley; Lewis Carter-Jones, whose major interest was the use of technology to aid the disabled; Fred Evans, the M.P. for Caerphilly and former headmaster of Pengam Grammar School, who, as the son of a Welsh miner, knew much about the hardships of the disabled from men injured in colliery accidents; Laurence Pavitt, chairman of the back-benchers health group and a sufferer from deafness who sat on the Medical Research Council; John Golding, the recently elected Labour M.P. for Newcastle-under-Lyme; and Arthur Latham.

Another Labour M.P., David Weitzman Q.C., was to give valuable help in drafting. He was a passionate supporter of the Bill.

On the Tory side, immediate interest was shown by such men as Neil Marten, a former junior minister and the chair-

man of the All-Party Disabled Drivers' Group; Maurice
Macmillan, son of the former Tory Premier; John Astor,
well known for his work for the disabled; James Prior,
Sir Clive Bossom, Dame Irene Ward and Sir Brandon
Rhys-Williams. Among leaders of voluntary organisations
who helped were Lady Hoare of the Society for Thalidomide
Children and Group Captain Leonard Cheshire V.C. of the
Cheshire Homes organization. Frank Price, the agent of the
Wythenshawe Labour Party also advised on details of the Bill.

The Bill was due for its Second Reading Debate on
Friday, 5 December. It was published with a week to spare
on 28 November. A few days before publication, Alfred
Morris gave a draft to David Ennals, Minister of State at the
Department of Health. He was surprised at the scope of the
Bill and had little time in which to consider the proposals.
Ennals promised Morris that for everything he had to take
out of the Bill, for whatever reason, he would put something
else in. Among four such items that the Government insisted
on taking out was a proposal to provide four-wheeled cars
for the disabled in place of the much criticized three-wheelers.
The Treasury threw up its hands in horror at the expense and
estimated that this item alone could cost £50 million.

The problems encountered by Alfred Morris in preparing
the Bill prompted the Commons Select Committee on
Procedure to call him to give evidence on the subject of
Private Members' legislation in March 1971. After he had
answered a number of inquiries about the difficulties he had
faced, Committee Member John Mackintosh, Labour M.P.
for Berwick and East Lothian, commented:

'It seems to me you have been too kind to everybody
all round. Am I correct in saying that when you took your
ideas to the departments chiefly concerned in the Government
none of them adopted the Bill as their own; you were left
to carry the burden of it and there was no suggestion that
they took it over from you or felt that you were doing
something they would have wanted to do? Am I right?'

Alfred Morris replied: 'There was no suggestion that they
should take the Bill over. It was put to me that a great deal of
extra work was involved in the propositions I was making.

I suppose there are people who feel that if their departmental affairs are to be the subject of a Private Member's Bill they ought to have thought of it first. But I would rather not say there was any resistance . . .'

This evidence to the committee was an important influence in bringing about proposals for reforms in the procedure to be adopted for such Bills.

The Government, in fact, might have decided to oppose the Bill on the grounds of its sheer size and cost. It had been hastily drafted and lacked detail. But some key members of the Government had already decided that it was a constructive measure and should be supported. They included the Chief Whip, Bob Mellish, as well as Fred Peart. These ministers worked behind the scenes to ensure that it had a fair run.

As the Bill grew in size, more and more Whitehall departments were drawn into the exercise. At the publication of the Bill, eleven ministries were already involved. Faced with this situation the Government was obliged to do some co-ordination behind the scenes. It was a Whitehall operation in co-ordination long overdue.

As Alfred Morris and his assistants worked on preparing the measure the major problem that emerged was that of identifying and registering the crippled and handicapped. There were only 235,000 disabled people on local authority registers. But the Disablement Income Group was saying that on the basis of considerable research there were some one and a half million. In fact, it was to emerge that there were several million adults in Britain outside hospitals who were suffering from some impairment – a physical or mental defect hampering them in their efforts to lead a normal life. About a third of those needed help ranging from assistance with some of the more tricky problems of dressing to constant care day and night. There were also thousands of disabled in hospitals and institutions and something like 100,000 handicapped children in England aged under sixteen.

Moreover, the number of disabled as a proportion of the population was and is growing. This is partly due to medical progress. More and more disabled babies are surviving.

Improved medical care also means that people suffering from disabling diseases are living longer. Better equipment and better diets are also increasing the survival rate. And people in general are living longer though they suffer from the impairments that come with old age.

The pace of modern living – both in business and on the road – is also adding to the total of disabled. In the executive suites middle-aged men are succumbing to a surfeit of heavy business lunches and crippling work pressures. On the roads, people are breaking themselves up in increasing numbers in high-speed crashes.

The pattern of disablement has changed with the increase in the numbers of disabled. The type of disablement resulting from motorway crashes – such as brain damage – is growing. The number of children with spina bifida – a congenital deformity of the bones forming the spinal column – is increasing, while polio and tuberculosis are no longer so prevalent. The biggest cause of impairment is arthritis. Something like three quarters of a million women and a quarter of a million men suffer from this crippling complaint. The most prevalent impairment connected with the central nervous system suffered by men results from cerebral haemorrhage. Men suffer more from coronary disease and lung disease resulting from their work in industry, while women suffer more from varicose veins, rheumatoid arthritis and migraine.

About a third of severely disabled people work, but the more typical disabled person is not of working age. The majority of disabled people want to work. Not only do they want to live as normally as possible; they need the money more than most. They need special foods and medical supplies. Their clothes need replacing more often than other people's due to the wearing effect of crutches and other support equipment. They often spend more on heating. But although they need work they are generally much slower at their jobs because of their disabilities and few can hope to earn a normal wage. For one reason or another, it is likely that no less than half the people who are badly incapacitated are living on the poverty line.

Living as they do on low pay or State benefits, it follows

that the standard of housing of the disabled is generally low too. A large proportion live in slum or semi-slum areas. Their social problems are enormous. Such are the difficulties of making an ordinary journey in terms of using public transport, access to buildings, use of public conveniences and the sheer expense, that many disabled people tend to live isolated, lonely lives. They have not been told to keep out of town halls, cinemas, theatres, art galleries, libraries and public conveniences, but they might just as well have been, for most of these buildings have been designed exclusively for the able-bodied.

The problem of mental handicap and deafness raises special difficulties for social intercourse. If a person is physically handicapped it will be apparent to neighbours who will often take a sympathetic and helpful interest. But if a person's impairment is mental, or if he is suffering from deafness, the neighbours will often assume that he is some sort of recluse who does not want to have social contacts.

This was the general scene as Morris and his friends and associates began work on their Bill. It was a situation in which hundreds of thousands who needed some sort of help were not known as individuals to their local authorities and sometimes not even to their neighbours. At best they were abstract statistics in some official's file, and as such received none of the aids to living that their condition entitled them to expect. The immediate issue was the difference between the numbers registered with local authorities and the minimum of one and a half million which the voluntary organizations estimated to be the true figure. The main problem therefore began to crystallize as that of finding the 'missing million'. It was a problem that began to catch the imagination of the press.

Within that broad problem, and behind the simplifying headlines of the newspapers were numerous other problems, problems almost as numerous as the disabled individuals themselves. They were the problems of care, housing, income, jobs, education and training, access, mobility, leisure . . . They were problems relating to every aspect of life in the twentieth century.

Chapter Two

~~~~~~

A Family Affair

MONICA, PRETTY but prematurely grey, is a thirty-year-old electronics worker in Lancashire. She looks after three disabled people – her mother, father and younger sister. Her mother suffers from rheumatoid arthritis which has destroyed her feet. Her father suffers from severe chronic bronchitis and has to sleep in the living room. Her sister is a mongol. She has another sister who lives nearby, but she suffers from a severe heart condition. Monica's mother has to be lifted in and out of bed. She can never go out alone and has to be given blanket baths. She sits all day in a wheelchair in her room while Monica is at work struggling to provide the family with an income. For this most severely disabled of households the local authority offered to provide a home help for only one hour on one day a week. Monica often asks herself how much it would cost the State if she were to break down and her father, mother and sister had to be put in institutions.

*   *   *

Mr M. was a graduate in his twenties working on a highly skilled communications project when he contracted multiple sclerosis, a disease of the nervous system, affecting arm and leg movement, sight and speech. Since 1966 he has been unemployed, confined to a wheelchair, unable to move his legs. He has to be fed, is incontinent, cannot see well enough to read and is completely dependent on other people. His wife, also a graduate, got herself a job for half the day so that she could take care of him. Because of her qualifications she earns a good salary even for part-time work. Nevertheless they spend well over the total of her income plus her husband's £6.55 a week allowance from the Department of Health and Social Security. The wife makes up the difference by working as a freelance journalist in the evenings.

Her day begins with a thirty-minute session of physiotherapy for her husband. She then gets her young daughter ready for nursery school and leaves the house at 7.45 a.m. From then until noon her husband is in a bed with cot sides to prevent him injuring himself. A home help visits twice a week for two hours for which they are charged by the local authority. The District Nurses arrive about noon to get the husband up, but once out of bed he cannot be left alone in case a spasm sends him slithering to the floor. Someone therefore has to be paid to help him from noon until Mrs M. arrives home at two o'clock. This service costs seven shillings an hour – and sometimes more if there are minor emergencies. Mrs M. collects her little girl from nursery school at about three o'clock and the rest of the afternoon is taken up by household chores, playing with the child and taking her husband out. Occasionally she must find time to collect items on prescription for her husband's incontinence and the pressure sores which he gets only rarely but which may take weeks to heal. After putting the child to bed Mrs M. does the household washing, sewing and repairs. She continually has to administer to her husband – move his legs, light his pipe, provide him with drinks. It takes an hour to get him ready for bed. Mrs M. is rarely in bed before midnight and sometimes has to work on a writing commission until the early hours. Finance is a very real problem. A car has become an essential but they have had to run it without assistance. If Mr M. were less disabled he would be eligible for a vehicle to drive himself. Another expense not allowed for by the authorities is the cost of proper feeding in such a case. If chair-bound people suffering from M.S. are not given a properly balanced diet they suffer from overweight, low physical condition, diarrhoea, boredom and depression.

Mrs P. of Hampshire was transformed by a stroke in 1964 from an active housewife to a near helpless invalid. Mr P. was advised to put her in a home and put their two children into care. He refused and for a time tried a number of compromise arrangements, including taking his baby daughter to work with him. Finally he decided to give up his £1,500-a-year job with its good prospects and company car and devote all his time to caring for his wife and running the home. They live on social security benefits which amount to about £18 a week. The hospital gave him a course in physiotherapy and he set about the slow but loving task of improving his wife's condition. After a year at home he was rewarded by some real and heartening progress. His wife had regained movement in her limbs and partially regained her speech. If he had left her in a hospital ward for geriatric patients – as he had been advised to do – she would have been a cabbage. As for Mr P.'s new life, it was not easy for him to leave his job and settle down to the household chores. But he says that it has made him realize just how important a woman's work is.

*   *   *

John Smith, twenty-six, is severely disabled and mentally retarded. He is unable to walk and an average day in his life consists of lying in bed until midday and then sitting strapped in his wheelchair doing jigsaw puzzles and watching television. He needs assistance for all his personal needs. He lives with his mother, who is divorced. Until recently she worked to provide a few extras to make life more tolerable for her son. But her mother, who lived with them and cared for John in the day, died in tragic circumstances and Mrs Smith had to give up her job to look after John. As a result she is now confined to the home day and night and relies on neighbours to do her shopping. She does not wish John to be sent to a residential home and the local Social Service Department has not been of much help. She has applied for an attendance allowance but it is doubtful whether anyone with experience will be found to care for John all day. The family's standard of living has slumped since Mrs Smith had to give up her job.

Millions of men, women and children who are not themselves disabled are affected by the problems of disability. They are part of families in which one or more members are handicapped. In fact a family that includes a disabled person becomes in a way a disabled household, subject to special problems, special hardships, special strains – and often special ties.

If the husband is disabled and unfit to work the family generally suffers from severe financial problems and a continual struggle to make ends meet. The man often gets despondent about his inability to provide for his wife and children. He will sometimes complain bitterly that he is no good to anyone, is on the scrap heap and would be better dead. He may resent being dependent on his wife and as a result their relationship will become strained and difficult. He may develop a guilt complex about his failure to give the children a good start in life. His depressions and bad temper will then tend to drive the children farther from him and increase his feeling of parental failure.   If the disabled husband is able to work he will almost certainly earn only a small wage – probably little more than he would receive from Social Security for sitting at home all day. The work may ease his pride and be good for his morale but financially the family will probably be little better off.

*   *   *

Mr B. is a middle-aged hemiplegic, suffering from paralysis on one side, who has worked for the same firm since leaving school. He does not earn very much. He walks with difficulty and depends on mechanical transport. He suffers from asthma, too, and frequently has to take time off because of his poor health. Sometimes he also has to take time off because of his wife's ill health. Her poor health has apparently been aggravated by the problems arising from her husband's disability. She has been a good wife and mother but has had a chronic depressive illness dating from the birth of her first child. It has become worse with succeeding pregnancies. Of the three children one has started work but two are still at school. Mr B. blames his disability for the restricted life the

family leads. He feels it has contributed a lot to his wife's ill
health. She is unable to go out alone and when she is badly
depressed he has to do all the household chores. Mr B. had
an invalid tri-car but although his wife is also handicapped
they are not eligible for a four-wheeled car through the
Health Department. A charitable organization gave them a
car several years ago and this made a great difference to the
well-being of the family. But the rising cost of living has faced
them with the prospect of having to sell the vehicle.

The family income is made up of Mr B.'s wages (£19 net
after deductions, including mortgage repayments), one
family allowance (90p), and a contribution from the earning
son of £3.60. The total weekly income is £23.50 of which
45 per cent is spent on food.

*   *   *

Mrs T., aged forty-eight, has four children, but only the two
eldest are normal. The third, aged fourteen, is a spastic girl;
the fourth, twelve, is an autistic boy. They live in a council
house in Dagenham. Mr T. deserted seven years ago. Mrs T.
has had big problems in finding suitable education for her
children. The boy has even been excluded from a local
authority special school because of his difficult behaviour.
Mrs T. has to cope with two severely handicapped children
and has no financial support. She is unable to leave either
child alone for more than a few minutes but her application
for an attendance allowance was turned down. She has been
unable to make many friends because of the demands of her
family. She has had no holiday for six years.

*   *   *

A moving account of the problems of nursing a disabled
husband has been written by Mrs Sylvia King of Bishops
Stortford for the Disablement Income Group Megan du
Boisson Memorial Prize. Mrs King, whose husband died of
multiple sclerosis in 1971 told her story – shortened for the
purpose of this book – in these words:

'Everything dated back to 1961. He had been in Greece

on his firm's behalf when he panicked because he thought himself unable to write easily . . .

'Several years passed with visits to physicians, neurologists and eye specialists – and there was no diagnosis! Meantime, the months passed with more and more frequent attacks of influenza and migraine, so called. As a family we suffered severely. No plans could be made that included Daddy unless they were provisional. Trips abroad on firm's business continued until 1964, but each one became more distressing and I can understand that the effort needed to take the responsibilities involved was excessive. There was always at least one episode of lethargy or sickness while he was away.

'What a vicious circle! When the firm realized that the burden was too great, and left him at his desk, the frustration was enormous and depression overshadowed everything else. Around this time, the methodical mind began to lose control. How can a perfectionist be satisfied with second-rate work? Rather than do something imperfectly things were left undone, always to be done tomorrow. (Looking through personal papers and files now I can trace this exactly.) Depression increased.

'We produced another child in 1966 to my delight, but that child knew from the moment he was born that there was trouble around him. He has always been the most demanding, yet most affectionate of the three children. He instinctively seemed to know that unless he insisted on my attention, he would not get a fair share of it. He has barely known his father, who died the week before he started school. For two and a half years, after my husband's premature retirement, the two of them battled for my constant attention. I am sure that my little son saved my sanity, as I had to be normal around the house and not get depressed myself. Now they are both gone within a week.

'The diagnosis established in 1967, we set about facing the future. I hinted that this illness must be fought, not accepted passively, but although he half understood this, it always seemed that he was waiting for the next day to arrive, when he would be feeling fitter. It was not until

about twelve months later, when he had lost ground, especially as regards speech and balance, that the same London
teaching hospital seemed to attempt to get a message
across. And then it was getting late to face facts; all effort
was needed to get up in the morning, face a day in the
office and literally exist in an armchair all evening.

'Perhaps the most difficult time for us all was in 1969,
when the Personnel Manager from my husband's firm
brought him home after a bad fall and announced that the
firm could no longer cope, or words to that effect. How
long he had been a "passenger" at the firm I never inquired. I had most carefully avoided such a topic of conversation with colleagues since I could guess that things
must be as bad there as at home. For some months prior to
this there had been ever-increasing episodes of loss of
balance and all the distress associated with this.

'With the final withdrawal from working life, a rapid
deterioration took place. I had feared this would happen.
No longer was it necessary to make an effort to get up each
morning and soon it was midday before he roused. The
incidence of falls increased and we never knew where we
would find him, but always it was the same picture – when
he fell he lay completely still with eyes shut as if to pretend
it had not happened. Great were my difficulties in getting
him up unaided and the harm this period did to the two
elder children cannot be judged.

'Having realized that the downhill slide was not to be
reversed, it occurred to me that a wheelchair was a neces-
sity. Now began a new phase of difficulties as we were in
touch with no one connected with equipment. Our doctor
arranged for an ambulance car to take us to the same
hospital as previously in order that a chair could be
ordered, but by the time the appointment came, it was impossible to get out to a car on two feet. This seemed an
insurmountable problem at the time.

'We then heard of the local Multiple Sclerosis Society
and it was a great relief to me to have two members pay us
a visit and to realize that there were other victims of M.S.
in our district . . .

'As time went on, many of our friends, though most sympathetic, gradually lost touch. Wives could chat to me when the occasion arose, but husbands found it so difficult to converse with someone who could barely make himself understood. It seldom occurred to former colleagues to come in small groups and just chat generally. One newly found local friend alone came regularly for the last twelve months and so kept up a continuity of small talk. How grateful I shall always feel for that.

'Despair I have felt so very often. Nobody can ever understand unless they have nursed a slowly declining husband, as I have done. Slowly the body systems ceased to function properly, but through it all the mathematical brain worked spasmodically on financial problems and gadgetry. How tragic it was when the voice was almost completely lost; I had to summon all my patience to get instructions into my unmathematical brain.

'Most of the time in the past twelve months, it would seem that there was no thought process, as there was little or no interest shown in things going on or in the children's progress, but obviously the brain power was only dulled, not diminished. We never discovered whether that depression that had been talked of so many years before was still a factor in the case.

'Yes, we had insurance to cover death, but not disablement. How many friends have taken note of our case and insured against disablement after seeing my husband's plight I do not know, but I do know it made many people stop and think on these lines. We were to consider ourselves lucky that he had been with one firm for twenty years. This firm was very fair to us and a pension of half-pay was something to be grateful for, as I was completely unable to earn anything myself, never having left the house for more than two hours for two years.

'I lost count of the number of forms I filled in over the years of disablement ... We watched the progress of the various government proposals to aid the chronic sick and disabled ... We joined D.I.G. last year and through its literature alone was I able to get a clear picture of government proposals for people with problems such as ours . . .

'Now I am alone with our three children, gradually putting the house back to its former state, before the dining-room had to become a bedroom, and wanting to think back to the years when we were a happy united family, though never forgetting the mental distress my husband suffered as a disabled person.'

Over a million impaired women in Britain are active house-wives, according to a government social survey published in 1971. Nearly half a million women living in their own homes cannot do most of their household chores because of their disabilities. For those who are able to do some housework the effort required is often very considerable. It takes a handi-capped woman much longer to do the chores and she tires more quickly. As a result she may become depressed and bad tempered.

Those confined to wheelchairs have the biggest difficulties in coping with the housework. Ordinary little jobs around the kitchen which a normal housewife does without effort be-come a nightmare for the disabled woman. Bending to clean the floor, reaching for items off shelves, lifting saucepans off the cooker . . . these are some of the most difficult problems facing her. Jobs that require a firm grip, such as opening tinned foods, can also present problems. Indeed, so much exhausting effort is required to prepare even a simple meal that many disabled people will go without when on their own – or rely on the local authority meals-on-wheels service.

General housework, too, presents difficulties connected with reaching, washing or moving heavy furniture. But the biggest problem for the disabled housewife is shopping. The mere effort of getting to the shops is bad enough for handi-capped people who have to rely on public transport. On top of that there are the problems of getting into shops that have stairs and narrow doors, queueing in restricted gangways, carrying heavy shopping bags.

Care of the children raises very special problems. And the mother who finds that she is unable to look after her children can become subject to tremendous emotional and psychological strains. The Government's 1971 survey estimates that there are some 76,000 impaired housewives living at home who have children under twelve. A large number encounter difficulties. Moreover, just as the disabled husband sometimes suffers from a feeling of guilt at his inability to provide for the family, so the handicapped mother may feel guilty of depriving her children of proper care and attention. Her inability to play with the children and to take them for treats to the cinema or the circus may add to her psychological problems. If she is in pain or depressed by frustrations she may become irritable and nag the children – with consequent feelings of remorse.

Mrs P. of Swansea, crippled with rheumatoid arthritis, interviewed for the *Western Mail*, said: 'I try to keep going even if the pain does make me a bit touchy sometimes. If I'm feeling a bit off and somebody drops something I really let fly at them, whoever it is. I wonder why my family put up with me sometimes.'

She has a son in his early teens whom she has never held, nursed or dressed. She had rheumatoid arthritis soon after he was born and could hardly move with it. She recalls: 'By the time I was able to wash him, dress and feed him, he was too old and could do all of that for himself. I still cry about that sometimes – I missed out on a lot of the pleasures most mothers get nursing their children.'

Here is a typical case history to illustrate the effect on the family if a member, such as the mother, becomes mentally ill: 'Mrs A. was a careful housewife and loving mother, who became irritable, anxious and depressed. She slowed down to such an extent that she could not finish her housework and maintain the high standards she set herself. Her husband was puzzled because she was no longer the companion she had been. The children never seemed to be able to please her – she was constantly finding fault and nagging. The youngest child started truanting from school and was referred to a child guidance clinic. When the family was consulted it was realized that the mother's illness was a contributory factor. She was advised to get help and fortunately she had enough understanding to see that she needed it.'

The more the wife is disabled the more the burden of running the home falls on the husband. Some manage to cope, aided perhaps by elder children, neighbours and home helps. Others find the strain too great and their own health breaks down, with disastrous effects on their own job and earning power.

Mr P. of Wales is married to a woman who is totally incapacitated by multiple sclerosis. For the past five years he has had to do everything for her. During that time he has had only two breaks – one of two weeks the other of five days. His health has been affected by overwork and his employers finally informed him that his domestic difficulties were affecting his efficiency. He has been reduced from his position as shop manager and transferred to another area as a salesman. He has been constantly urged by his doctor to send his wife to an institution but has always refused. He has thus saved the State thousands of pounds. Yet when he applied for an attendance allowance this was refused.

Sometimes the husband decides to give up his own job and devote himself full-time to caring for his wife and family at home. This is a big and difficult step to take. The decision to exist on State aid for the remainder of one's life is not one that comes easily to most men. It involves a big drop in income for most families if the man is able bodied and has been employed full-time. Sometimes a man will retire early on a small pension and in this type of case hardship can be just as great as State aid is reduced accordingly.

Mr P. of London retired early from the police after twenty-six years to care for his wife who has been almost totally disabled for ten years with multiple sclerosis. In 1970, when they were both in their early fifties, his pension was just over £11 a week. He buys out of that a non-employed National Insurance stamp, costing about £1. If he did not own his own house he would not know how to manage. From nearly £30 a week he has dropped to only about £10. Their living standards have plummeted. He writes: 'No car now – only a wheelchair to push my wife about in when the weather permits. No holidays for us and no help from anybody. What little capital I had has been slowly dwindling when bills for house repairs come in. We hear a lot about welfare services yet we've never seen a welfare officer. In fact, we are forgotten.'

Chapter Three

~~~~~~

The Child

A BOY'S body was found floating in the River Stour in the autumn of 1971. He was seven when he died. But he had the mentality of a six-week old baby. He had been unable to walk or talk and had no sense of balance. His father, charged with murder, made a statement which the defending lawyer described as 'one of the saddest documents I have ever seen . . . ' That statement described the anguish of loving parents who had lost all hope as their child became steadily worse. The little boy's fits had become more frequent and he developed screeching noises. The man explained: 'My wife tried so hard. It was terrible to watch her struggling so hard with him.'

The child was taken regularly to a local hospital. One day his mother wrapped him tenderly in a fur coat and his father took him for yet more treatment. But when he got there he realized that the little boy was much worse than any of the other patients at the hospital. He decided that he could not leave the child there. He started to drive home but on the way he stopped the car and carried his son to a brook. Gently he laid him in the water. The little boy drifted slowly away. The father explained later: 'I knew my son was at rest.'

*   *   *

Belinda Rothwell of Tottenham was eight years old when they removed her leg. She had started to complain about a pain eight months earlier. The doctors said it was 'psychosomatic'. In January 1971 Belinda collapsed from pain and was taken to the local hospital. 'I couldn't believe what was happening,' her mother told journalist Peta Van den Bergh of the *Hornsey Journal*. 'I was shown the X-ray of her leg. The doctor told me it was cancerous, and I broke down.' A day later she was begging the doctors to remove the leg. She recalled later: 'I stood there crying and saying that I wouldn't let her die. I thought that she might be saved if they took the leg off. They told me they would only do that as a last resort.' Despite intensive radio-therapy treatment it finally came to that.

Belinda knew something was very wrong. Her mother said: 'I didn't tell her at the beginning. I couldn't. I used to ask her if she knew that people sometimes had new legs. Then one day she asked me if she was going to have the leg off.' Her mother gently broke the news, explaining to the little girl that a new leg would prevent the cancer spreading. This knowledge and the terrible pain from which the child was suffering were not the only difficulties the mother had to face. She was unmarried and lived in a house for unmarried mothers. Her only money was a social security payment and her financial problems started the first time Belinda went into hospital.

'We all shared a telephone and one day it rang at three in the morning. I thought: "Oh God, it must be Belinda." Thankfully it wasn't.' But Miss Rothwell realized then that she would have to get her own phone. It took countless visits to the Welfare Department and finally to her M.P., Norman Atkinson, before she was provided with one. When the bill arrived for installation she was given a loan from the mayor's fund to pay for it.

The six months that Belinda was at home before the operation were 'unbelievable'. She couldn't travel on public transport – it hurt too much. 'I used to take her about in taxis. We couldn't go to any parks or cinemas because it hurt her and because there were steps.' Then the hospital told her to take Belinda away on holiday and 'build her up' before the operation. 'I couldn't afford to,' explained Miss Rothwell. 'I hadn't got any money at all. Then the hospital welfare department gave me money for the fare to take Belinda up to my family in Middlesbrough. I couldn't tell the hospital that they lived in worse conditions than we do here. But we went up.'

Belinda went back to hospital in September for her operation. After her leg had been amputated she didn't complain at all. If anyone asked her about it she replied: 'It's been blown away in the wind.' She was told she would be fitted with an artificial limb in about two months. But this raised new problems for her mother. She had to find some way of getting more living space. In her flat she shared a tiny bedroom with Belinda and there was not enough space to store the limb and fix up the balance bars the child would have to use. They also shared a kitchen and bathroom with other occupants of the house. As 1972 opened they were still waiting for a larger flat . . .

* * *

Peter is seven – a severely handicapped spastic, mentally and physically. He is totally dependent on others and needs washing, dressing and feeding. He gets around by rolling on the floor. He is blind, has no speech and is subject to fits. The whole house revolves round him. He attends a special school daily. His father is a chemist and his mother has suffered from a severe heart condition since his birth. He had an older sister Mary who died of cancer after a long illness, and his older brother John is ten. At times John has to mind, lift and generally assist his mother with Peter. Although John is an intelligent boy he is a year behind with his school work and his mother feels that he needs much more of her time – time she is physically unable to give him. Peter occasionally spends two weeks in a small Family Help unit and when he is away John is a different boy. The family have been offered a permanent hospital place for Peter. But despite the effect his continued presence at home is having on his mother's health and his brother's progress Peter's father feels unable to accept the offer.

* * *

There are estimated to be about 100,000 handicapped children in Britain under the age of sixteen. This is only a rough estimate – made by the Government. Children were not included in the Government's survey of the handicapped and impaired published in May 1971 – for technical reasons. Some people would say that there are good technical reasons for another survey to produce with some urgency concrete facts and figures about the growing number of disabled youngsters in the United Kingdom. The number of children with disabilities – and with several disabilities – is growing because advances in medicine have led to a higher survival rate among children at birth. The large number of children injured in road accidents adds to the annual toll.

The pattern of disablement among children has also changed over recent years and will continue to change as progress in research produces the means to prevent and cure certain diseases or to enable children born with severe handicaps to live. By the late 1960s cerebral palsy – a paralysis due to abnormal development or damage to the brain – had risen to first place as the chief cause of handicap among children. Spina bifida – a congenital deformity of the spine causing paralysis from the waist down – had also risen. Heart disease, which had once been the most common disablement, had dropped to third place. And there had been a big drop in the number of cases of polio.

Cerebral palsy is a condition in which a person has difficulty in making certain movements due to a fault in the brain at a time when it was still developing – which means before the child was three or four years old. One type of cerebral palsy is known as spastic – a word derived from spasm. This condition should strictly speaking refer to an unusual stiffness in the muscles. But as most children with cerebral palsy suffer from some muscular stiffness anyway, the word spastic has become synonymous with cerebral palsy.

A spastic child is born in Britain every eight hours. There are about 100,000 spastics in the country of whom about 7,000 are under the age of five. Many spastic children have only a slight handicap and can cope with life without too much difficulty. The Emperor Claudius, who as a young man was a butt of the Roman court because of weak legs and a speech impediment, was probably a spastic. At the other extreme some spastics cannot move at all and everything has to be done for them.

For centuries spastics were written off as strange cripples and idiots. Many have been shut away in institutions in this century. But if a spastic child has treatment very early – preferably from babyhood – there is a chance that he may be able to walk and run like other children.

Because so little was being done by the authorities to help spastics, the Spastics Society was formed in 1952. Under the directorship of James Loring it seeks to promote treatment and care of spastics, to help their families and to promote research into the causes, prevention and treatment of cerebral palsy.

The increase in spina bifida – which literally means split spine – is a good example of the way in which a new disablement suddenly appears to emerge to the public as a result of medical advance. The disability occurs when the spinal bones are not properly formed while the baby is in the womb. Many babies disabled in this way are also affected by hydrocephalus – water on the brain – which occurs when there is an obstruction to the circulation of the cerebrospinal fluid. But a treatment has now been devised which enables children to overcome even quite severe initial hydrocephalus, and surgeons have discovered a method of operating on the spine which has also added to the survival rate: now about fifty per cent compared to less than ten per cent a few years ago. But the children who survive, although they often enjoy normal intelligence, are usually paralysed below the waist and face life in a wheelchair with problems of incontinence. The problems are such, in fact, that there has been some argument in medical circles about the extent to which attempts should be made to save the most serious cases. Should they be allowed to die? Where should the line be drawn, ask these medical men, with a detachment that the parents could never share?

There is a wave of spina bifida children just coming up to school age and many schools are not yet equipped to cope with them, especially in the provision of lavatories. The number of cleft-spine babies born in South Wales is more than double the average for the whole of Britain. Research is now under way to discover why the incidence should be so heavy in that part of the country and whether this is connected with some element in the local environment. The incidence in South Wales is 4·7 per thousand and in parts of North Monmouthshire the rate is nearly seven per thousand. As a result of a local-based charity named TENOVUS, Cardiff Royal Infirmary had the first fully-equipped sterile spina bifida unit in the world. As soon as the disease is detected at the birth of the child it has to be transferred to sterile surroundings to prevent further infection.

On the general problem of disability among children, Medical Officers of Health have been notifying the Government since the mid 1960s of all cases of congenital malformations observed at birth. This relatively new practice has produced an overall rate of about 16 per 1,000 births.

It is usually an appalling shock to parents to discover that they have a disabled child. It can put tremendous strains on the family. First reactions can be of misery, despair and guilt.

Mr and Mrs W. have been married for about eight years and had five children in quick succession. Mr W. is very sensitive about the fact that he is illiterate. He probably hoped for compensation in a perfect son. But Keith, the eldest child, was born disabled. Mr W. lived in hope that his wife would produce a son not handicapped or backward in any way. However, the next four children were girls. Now the physical relationship between Mr and Mrs W. has deteriorated until it has become repellent to the wife.

*　　*　　*

Mary was born weak and very jaundiced. She did not feed well and soon started fits. The Infant Welfare doctor repeatedly assured the parents that there was nothing wrong with the child. But the mother became increasingly agitated and felt she was inadequate. She became depressed and was put on drugs. After much insistence by the parents, Mary was referred to a famous children's hospital. There a consultant told the parents that the child had suffered from brain damage since birth and that nothing could be done for her. Now at four years of age Mary cannot sit and cannot hold anything. She is totally dependent on her parents and suffers from fits. In the last year or two she has cried incessantly at night. The strain has been so great on the parents that both have been put on drugs. Mary has been admitted to hospital for short term care to give her mother and father the opportunity of a good night's sleep. A second child, a little boy aged three, has become increasingly difficult to handle. This is because Mary requires so much attention. The little boy has also started to resent his sister's presence after her absence for a time in hospital. He was so jealous at one time that it was not safe to leave the children alone together. The mother has become more and more despairing and irritable. At times she has felt like leaving the whole family.

*   *   *

It would be wrong to give the impression that a disabled child in the home automatically means unhappiness and discord. On the contrary, a handicapped child can help to cement a marriage and bring much happiness to parents, brothers and sisters.

Mrs B. of Sussex, in a letter to the Central Council for the Disabled about her two-year-old spastic child, wrote: 'I want you to know how dear she is to us . . . how her brothers and sisters want to keep her . . . Our eldest boy won a school prize recently for being the most helpful and considerate child in the school. So perhaps she has taught them a little consideration for others . . . '

That letter was written after the family had suffered a rebuff from the local authority to a request for a ramp so that the child's wheelchair could be pushed easily over some awkward steps leading into the garden. Mrs B. after undergoing a stomach operation, found the effort of lifting the wheelchair over the steps half-a-dozen times a day too much for her. But she was told by the local Borough Engineer that it would be too expensive for the council to put a ramp over the steps. The local Health Visitor told her: 'Don't waste the town's money – put the child away.'

*   *   *

For the disabled child the prospect is so often one of deprivation, struggle and disappointment. He wants and needs to be like other children. Yet he may be unable to walk or run, use his arms or legs, or even sit upright. The disabled child will probably spend much of his time indoors. He will often be lonely. And as his parents try to make up for his disabilities with special care and attention he may become self-centred and preoccupied with his own problems.

Because a handicapped child tends to get extra attention from parents other children in the family can become resentful. A Sussex woman who has a sister who is mentally handicapped has recalled the strains this caused in her childhood.

'At first my parents thought she was backward and she was sent to a special school. My mother brought her home for the holidays. I can remember when I was about six or seven never really being able to look forward to school holidays at home because she would be there, and also resenting the fact that I would be punished for doing something while she was let off scot free for doing the same thing, or worse. Parents may think they should devote more of their time to their handicapped child but that is like penalizing the others because they are normal. That's how I felt when I was a child . . . '

Holiday time can be a particularly trying time for families with a disabled child. The following account of holiday problems for a family with a spastic child was given at a conference a few years ago.

'In families like mine holidays are looked forward to each year just as much as in other families. Why then do they fall a little flat? Is it the continual lifting of wheelchair and child, in and out of the car? Is it always having to find a beach with a minimum of steps or a slope down to it? Or is it that once on the beach, pushing a wheelchair on soft sand can be a nightmare? One must remember that this is a handicapped child's holiday, too, so any request from the child to go in the sea must be fulfilled if possible, either by mummy or daddy or both. For the child who cannot even stand up this means lifting the child out of the chair, undressing him, putting him in his bathing suit, carrying him down to the sea, holding him whilst in the sea, carrying him out again, drying and dressing him. As the holiday progresses this can become very tiring.

The comment must often be passed: "Is it worth it?" But of course it is – for the child's sake anyway. Many parents of children who can partially walk return home from a holiday tired and with strained backs. It is not easy for a father to squash a child's enthusiasm for a walk on the promenade, even though he knows that he will probably have to carry the child back. I have talked to parents of teenage spastics and they admit that they have never really had a holiday since the child was born.'

Not unnaturally much emphasis has been placed over the years on trying to help disabled children cope with their disabilities. But this has often led to neglect of the disabled boy or girl's needs as a child. There is now a growing feeling that the disabled child should be allowed to integrate as much as possible in normal life. Some experts warn, however, that too much talk of integration can be an illusion. They argue that it is important to prepare handicapped children for a life of dependence rather than independence.

In the field of education, the move towards integration has led to the belief that the disabled child should be helped to become part of the ordinary school system. The first National Conference of the Joint Council for the Education of Handicapped Children was held in Manchester in July 1970. Mr L. Bowstead, President of the Association for Special Education, summing up the discussions, reflected a widely held view that, while there were always likely to be children, so severely handicapped that they could not be educated in ordinary schools without detriment to themselves and others, there were many others with milder handicaps, now in special schools, who could be educated in ordinary schools if they were suitably staffed and equipped.

The point was made at the conference that it should be compulsory for all local authorities to ensure early detection of handicaps in a child and provide appropriate special educational guidance and treatment. The very early need of parents for special help and advice should be recognized by the authorities. Infant and primary-school teachers should be suitably trained in observing and recording in the early school years, and short screening procedures should be used on a wide scale to detect handicaps that had gone unnoticed.

The first children provided with special schools in Britain were the blind and the deaf. Later on schools were set up for crippled children and those with mental disabilities. In more recent years special schools have been opened for spastics, children suffering from spina bifida, and those handicapped by autism and communications difficulties. But special schools raise a problem. The more specialized they are the wider the area from which they must draw their pupils. This means that the children often have to attend as boarders and there is thus added to their disability the extra problem of being removed from parents and friends. Boarding schools can of course ease the pressures on families. But the removal of the child can also add to the parents' feelings of inadequacy. Sometimes they will refuse to send their child . . .

George is a ten-year-old spastic, disabled to the point where he can only walk with considerable difficulty and needs help with small clothing items such as buttons and laces. His words are few and very indistinct. But he can use his hands and feed himself. The local authority suggested that he should start his education at the village school but his parents decided that this was not the answer as he was unable to defend himself and they feared he would be harmed by the more boisterous children. He has a normal I.Q. and the county has no school for the physically handicapped appropriate for him. He has been attending a junior training centre in a nearby town but the staff are concerned because he is not receiving the type of education and stimulation he needs. A place has been offered in a Spastics Society school but the parents do not want him to go to a residential school as they are a closely knit family. It may well be that George will not have the opportunity of sheltered or perhaps open employment which would have been available if he had received appropriate education.

The difficulties facing a disabled child who attends an ordinary school are numerous. Susan, aged fifteen, was born with both hips dislocated and can only get around by using walking sticks. She goes to the local high school and encounters all sorts of problems. The mere task of carrying her books from class to class is one. Her parents have tried various solutions including a duffle bag but the ropes bruised her shoulders. Travelling to school presents another problem. The staff of the local railway station have refused to help carry her up and down to the platform. The medical authorities recommended swimming as a regular exercise to ease her condition – but the local authority failed to make regular arrangements.

The autistic child faces special problems. Autism, first diagnosed only in the 1940s, is an inability to communicate – an impairment in the development of language, through speech, writing or gesture. Because of this communication problem, autistic children tend to live in a world of their own and often become very difficult to handle. They can go berserk and scream and rampage for long periods.

Statistical surveys have suggested that four or five children out of every 10,000 of school age are autistic. Until recently they were classed with the mentally handicapped. But many autistic children are of average or above average intelligence. Hundreds are in mentally sub-normal units who should not be there. In any case, most institutions for the mentally handicapped lack the staff and equipment to enable them to help autistic children reach their full potential. The National Society for Autistic Children is now doing much to call attention to the plight of these children and to get the type of specialized education they need.

Lady Ruthven, who has worked in psychiatric hospitals and has seen a large number of autistic children, has told the House of Lords of the extraordinary difference between the treatment given now and what was done some years ago. 'I have a friend who has an autistic son. He went to school but not to a school for autistic children. This boy is now twenty-two. He had some fits in adolescence and has deteriorated a good deal since then. He is now in a closed ward in hospital for his aggressive behaviour . . . at the moment he is on large doses of tranquilizers. I compare him with a little boy I know of eight or nine in a hospital in the area where I worked. He is a nice little boy, with a high I.Q., but he is very aggressive. Before he came to us he had been in a big London hospital where I believe he caused damage amounting to at least £2,000. We had a padded cell built for him and he had to have four nurses, because he had not only damaged everything he could damage but had also hurt himself and could not be allowed with other children. The last time I saw him, after he had been seen by a great authority on autistic children who advised certain treatment, he was with three other people in the dining room of the hospital, talking to his nurse. He was not quite intelligible. I could understand only a word or two of what he was saying but the nurse obviously understood everything he said.

'So I should like to say there is a chance for all autistic children if they are found and diagnosed at an early stage, are given the proper education, taken to the right places . . . '

Serious education and employment problems exist for another group of children who suffer from the disability known as dyslexia – a condition which some educational psychologists refuse to admit exists. It is applied here to children who suffer from special reading difficulties although there is nothing wrong with their eyes or their intelligence. It is popularly known as word blindness. There are no official statistics of the complaint.

Dyslexic children attending an ordinary school do not usually fall into any clear category for the teacher. They often have a high intelligence and a desperate longing to learn. Failure to make headway can sometimes change the personality of such a child. He may become anti-social and turn to crime. A high percentage of young offenders are non-readers. The big problem arises when the youngster tries to get a job. A dyslexic boy has explained how his teachers have not understood him. 'They just thought I was lazy. I've told them I wanted to learn but I don't think they believed me. I would like to have been a teacher myself. But now I've got to find a job that I can do without reading or writing. That means manual work.'

Children who are both deaf and blind present another very special problem – and one for which few local authorities have made special provision in the past. One reason for this is that deaf-blindness occurs only sporadically. But the education problem can be appreciated from this explanation: if a child is completely blind but only partially deaf he is likely to be sent to a school for the blind where the teacher will be unable to cope with the deafness. If, however, the child is completely deaf and only partially blind then the teacher trying to use lip-reading methods of instruction will not be able to cope with a child suffering from defective eyesight.

Many disabled children, for one reason or another, end up as long-stay patients in hospitals. There were 7,000 mentally handicapped youngsters and 1,500 physically handicapped to whom hospital was home in 1971. In the recent past some of these youngsters have been placed in geriatric wards, where the atmosphere of senility and near death has had an appalling effect on them.

An important gap in the law with regard to children who live in hospitals has been publicised by Maureen Oswin of the National Association for the Welfare of Children in Hospital. She has pointed out to the Government that there is nothing in the Children's Acts to say that the standard of 'home care' for such youngsters should be equal to the standard of care given to a child who is put in a foster home. That means that long-stay hospital children can live in very poor conditions that would never be tolerated in a foster home. For example, they do not have regular holidays or outings, they lack personal belongings or clothes or places to keep their toys; they do not have their own housemother; they have no privacy and undergo mass bathing and toilet routines . . .

Maureen Oswin has pointed out that there would be a public outcry if a local authority was found to be looking after children in such poor conditions.

The case of Albert sums up the need: he is twenty-six, mentally handicapped, and has lived in a hospital since he was six years old. His entire childhood and youth have been spent in a crowded ward with between thirty and forty other handicapped people. He has had no locker and nowhere to put his belongings or hang photos. He has never had the pleasure of seeing food cooked and has rarely sat at a properly laid table. As a little child he never knew the security of a house mother. Albert, not surprisingly, is shy and awkward. He has led an excessively deprived life for more than twenty years – and he is likely to continue to do so for many more to come.

Chapter Four

~~~~~~

Earning a Living

IN JUNE 1970 an unemployed father drawing only £11 a week social security was jailed in England for fifty days because he could not pay a £16 fine imposed on two of his three sons. He had been made responsible by the court for paying the fine because the boys were under fourteen years of age. The man, in his mid-forties, had been unemployed for five years due to chronic sickness. Whenhe had last worked he had been employed as a railway shunter and because his wages had been so low he was 'wage stopped' by the Supplementary Benefits Commission and was drawing in social security £3.50 less than the poverty level set for a man with his family commitments. (The wage stop is the system by which people are prevented from drawing more in State benefits than they earned while in work. This iron law is applied even if it means that a family then has less to live on than the Supplementary Benefit Commission's own officially recognized poverty line.)

The man had applied to the local office of the Department of Health and Social Security for help in paying his fine. He was flatly refused. His sons had been accused of stealing golf clubs from a car abandoned on a scrap heap. The detectives on the case took the boys' shoes away for examination. They were the only shoes possessed by the boys. They went without while the police carried out their inquiries.

*   *   *

In the City of Exeter in 1970 a family of four, three of

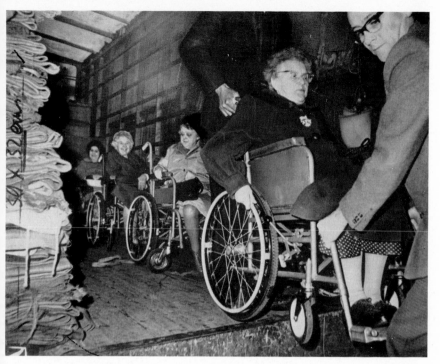

Disabled women being unloaded from a furniture van that takes them every month from their homes to a tea and concert organized by the local Cripples' Guild.

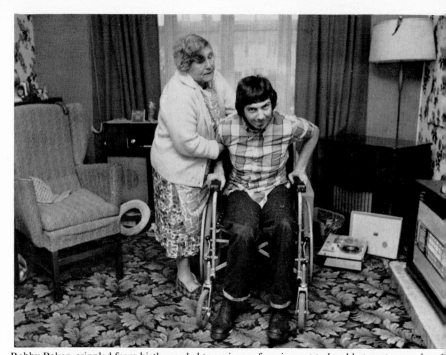

Bobby Baker, crippled from birth, needed two pieces of equipment to be able to get around on his own at home – a ramp for the front door and rails inside the house. For three years his widowed mother asked Hillingdon Borough Council to make the adaptations to her council house at West Drayton, Middx. When action was taken after this long delay she was asked to pay part of the cost although she had eight other children and found it far from easy to make ends meet.

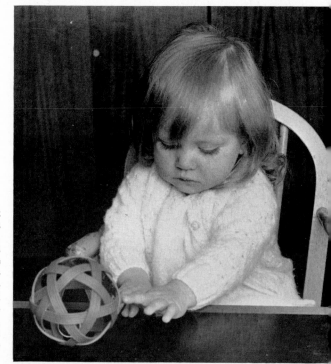

Sally Anne Rampton, at sixteen months, reaches for her toy. In vain. Sally cannot see. This picture was taken at the Child Development Research Unit, Nottingham, where Sally and other handicapped children play with toys, watched by staff from behind a panel of 'one-way' glass.

whom were disabled, were existing on a weekly income of £20.62. The disabled father, a man of great independence of mind, insisted on trying to cope with a full-time job rather than fall back on State assistance. The family found life a constant struggle – a struggle made more difficult by a house totally unequipped for disabled people. The whole house and water were heated by one open fire and the family had been waiting ten months for an immersion heater to be fitted. After paying tax and insurance the father was left with £17.23 to cover the rent of £4.26, diet and prescription costs for the three disabled people, and the normal living costs of four.

* * *

A war pensioner wrote this letter in 1970 to the Central Council for the Disabled:

'When it comes to seeking some light part-time employment to supplement my income this is no joke. To tell any employer in this area that you are a registered disabled person is like signing your own death certificate. In January 1970, owing to my disability, I had to go into hospital for a general check-up, with promises galore from my employer of my job always being safe, and that I had no fear of not having a job to come back to. I had been in hospital for five days when my wife received by post my insurance cards and income tax form. I had been dismissed – not even a letter giving me a week's notice or any pay. I was dismissed because I was ill and disabled.

'I do not ask for charity in any shape or form, but just a chance to do a job of work, and this requires employers to relent and say "Yes" when people like myself apply for a job instead of giving the same answer all the time, which is "No." '

* * *

Katherine Andres was hurrying to get rations to the British troops in Aden after curfew in 1966 when she was shot in the face and back by Arab terrorists. As a result she is paralysed from the armpits down and is likely to remain so for the rest of her life. She cannot sit upright unless she is supported by special corsets. But she has now got the use of her hands and has been taught to type again. She would make an excellent secretary as she is very active when in her wheelchair. But by 1971 Katherine had become very depressed by the lack of response to her advertisements in the newspapers. Despite a great deal of pressure on the Government she has been awarded no compensation on the ground that she was employed in Aden by a private contractor. Yet if she had been shot and paralysed in Britain by a criminal she would have been eligible for compensation. She needs accommodation and work – and if these were provided she would be able to leave hospital where a bed would be freed and the Exchequer would be saved at least £40 a week.

*   *   *

Mr B. was married with two children when he was disabled by polio. It left him paralysed in both legs, with very limited use of his arms, and incapable of driving even an invalid tricycle. At the time he and his wife owned a small car and she was able to drive him and the children. But shortage of money forced them to give up the car – and shortage of money was a major factor in the break-up of their marriage. Mr B. is now living at public expense in a home for the disabled.

*   *   *

Miss W., a mentally ill, depressed woman, was pensioned off from her fairly high-level job on medical grounds. She was unable to keep up the mortgage repayments on her house and severe depression led to an over-dose of drugs and admission to hospital. When the hospital had dealt with this immediate illness it gave her two days' notice of discharge, although her personality problems were as acute as ever. She had no job and nowhere to live. After some pressure the hospital agreed to keep her until some housing was found. A room was provided in a small private hotel – an unsatisfactory arrangement – and she has since had to cope with trying to find a job. She continually seeks to solve her problems of finance, employment and housing by taking another over-dose in order to be re-admitted to hospital.

*   *   *

Most disabled people who work are unable to do as much or earn as much as a person who is not handicapped by a disability. The rate of unemployment among disabled people is far higher than the general level. In fact, it has generally exceeded the national jobless figure by four or five times. Yet work is of tremendous importance to the disabled. It is important for their standard of living; also for their pride and self-respect. It is important for their health, both physical and mental, and from the point of view of social contact. There is another aspect too. The more disabled people are able to work, the more they will be able to contribute to the national wealth and the less they will have to rely on State assistance. But the majority of disabled people are, in fact, beyond working age – a state of affairs that should perhaps remind us that potentially we are all disabled.

There are only about 700,000 impaired men and women in the national work force. About half of them are skilled or semi-skilled manual labourers. Of the 74,000 more severely disabled in jobs, some four out of ten complain that their disability has forced them into work in which their qualifications are not used. Thus, to the burden of their handicap is added the frustration and heartbreak of failing to get work in line with their ability.

Mary Greaves, the Honorary Director of the Disablement Income Group, who has made a study of the employment problems of disabled people, has summed up the situation as one of fitting a minority group into an environment designed for a majority group.

'If everyone were blind there would be no problem in not being able to see; man would create an environment where lack of sight was a disadvantage of the same order as not being able to fly.'

The fact that the disabled are a minority group with special employment problems has been recognized by the State for some years. The Disabled Persons Employment Acts of 1944 and 1958 provide the legislative framework: a Disabled Persons Register and an obligation on firms employing twenty people or more to employ at least three per cent from that register.

To be eligible to get on the register a person must be substantially handicapped, be prevented from obtaining work suited to his qualifications and have a reasonable chance of being employed. Once a person is on the register he is eligible for admission to a retraining unit and help in finding a job.

The register is far from comprehensive. There has been no attempt to compel people seeking work to register and any attempt would be strongly resisted by the handicapped. As a result it does not include all those who are employed nor all those unemployed who would like a job. It is often the most severely disabled who are the most reluctant to register. At times of high unemployment handicapped people are even less likely to register as they suspect that there can be no prospect of work for them. From long experience they know that the handicapped are usually the first to be made redundant when firms are cutting down on staff. Those capable of only light work are usually the most vulnerable and the first to go when economies are being made. A levy like the Selective Employment Tax also makes firms less inclined to employ disabled people. The register, in fact, far from being able to cope with the problem of unemployed disabled people is a useful guide to the incidence of unemployment among them. In the spring of 1970 it revealed that unemployment was as high as 11.36 per cent. By mid 1971 the number of unemployed among the employable disabled was five times the national average. By March 1972 the proportion of registered who were unemployed had soared to 14·9 per cent.

Registration reached its peak in 1950 when 900,000 people were listed. This was no doubt due partly to the large number of disabled ex-servicemen and also to the wartime habit of complying with invitations to register. But the number of registered had dropped by nearly a third between 1950 and 1970.

What of the linked legislation obliging firms with twenty or more workers to employ three per cent of disabled? The truth is that many large firms come nowhere near to fulfilling their quota. In 1971 about half the employers were dodging their obligation. Meanwhile over half the disabled in work were employed by firms with less than twenty workers. Some

were employed by firms using them to make profits out of
door-to-door sales rackets. It has been estimated that at least
forty firms in Britain were involved in this racket in 1971.
They operated by employing a small number of handicapped
people on small wages and using slick door-to-door salesmen
to give housewives the impression that they represented
registered charities. The goods sold are often shoddy, such as
manufacturers' rejects that could not be sold on their own
merits. Firms running the racket register under the Trading
Registrations (Disabled Persons) Act 1958, and take on
disabled people for a short time while doing so. Once registered they often get rid of a number of handicapped people
until it is time to register again with the Department of
Employment.

A large number of disabled people say they have had
trouble at some time in getting work because of their handicaps. Not only are they usually limited in the type of work
they can do. They also have to face up to the fact that they
cannot work at the same pace as non-disabled people and
tire more quickly.

David, twenty-four, is disabled to the point where he is
unable to stand for long periods and the use of his right hand
is so restricted that he cannot easily use hand tools. He comes
from a working-class family and attended a secondary
modern school where he got average results. On leaving
school he worked as a post boy in a local factory office, but
eventually it was found that he was unable to cope and he
was asked to leave. Since then he has attended a rehabilitation
centre and has had several operations in hospital. His
physical condition has deteriorated sharply in recent years –
and this is partly due to depression and lack of work. He is
very lonely, withdrawn and self-conscious. His morale has
suffered greatly because he has been unable to find a job.

Press accounts of disabled people holding down key posts
are sometimes misleading. Social workers explain that often in
such cases the disabled person does not do a full day's work
and is subsidised in some way. This can be a severe blow to
the pride of a disabled person anxious to prove that he is
independent and as good as the next man. The discovery

that this is not so can pile psychological problems on top of the physical disability. The feeling of being an outsider – not part of the team – is accentuated, too, in firms where handicapped people are barred from joining the pension scheme. The work problem becomes particularly acute for people with certain types of disabilities that embarrass or scare their fellow workers. This is the case, for instance, with epileptics. Their fits tend to frighten or worry colleagues, and some employers will not employ them for that reason. There are cases, however, of colleagues covering up for epileptics when they have fits to protect them from getting the sack. The problem for the epileptic is brought out in a letter from a girl in her mid twenties who had been unemployed for fifteen months and was finding great difficulty in getting work. She can do a good day's work if only given the chance. But a few hours after being interviewed for a post and getting the job she received a letter from the person who had been prepared to take her on. It read: 'I hate having to write this letter but I am afraid I have to say that we cannot offer you the job after all. This is not because we don't want you, for we all took to you very much, but simply because of the epilepsy. I have had a talk with Miss X. and she gave you a wonderful reference but explained about your bad luck in having these fits . . . ' The girl had not told them about her health. She was desperate for a job.

Sheltered workshops have been set up by the Government, local authorities and voluntary organizations to provide people with work who are too handicapped to get a job in 'open' or normal industry. The most famous organization operating in this field is Remploy Ltd, an independent, subsidised company set up following the 1944 Act. Remploy has some 85 factories all over Britain employing a total of over 7,500. The average weekly wage for Remploy workers in 1971 was about £15. But it was making on average a loss of about £9 per worker per week.

A National Advisory Council on the Employment of the Disabled operates to assist the Secretary of State for Employment on the problem of training and employing handicapped people. The Employment Ministry has over a thousand officials called Disablement Resettlement Officers working throughout the country to assist disabled people seeking jobs. These officials often come in for much praise from the disabled people they help but the system under which they operate has attracted some sharp criticism. The complaint is made, for instance, that the officers spend only part of their careers in this field and therefore fail to build up the experience and specialized knowledge needed to do a proper job. Their offices are often poked away in attic-like accommodation inaccessible to disabled people. The point is made, too, that they do not cater for professional people.

A young woman who was considered too disabled for manual work inquired, for instance, whether there was some suitable job, if possible of a literary nature. She was given no helpful advice at all. Indeed, she was told that her best course was to go on the dole. After making inquiries in other quarters she enrolled for a course arranged by the London School of Journalism and as a result of that course she obtained employment. But it was only after she reported to the D.R.O. that she had got a job that she was told that there was a course in journalism available through the Department of Employment.

A young man in his mid-twenties, holding O levels in mathematics and book-keeping, complains that because he is a spastic he has had to find employment in a spastics workshop cutting firewood and doing similar odd jobs.

A registered disabled man, suffering from muscular dystrophy – a progressive wasting of the muscles – complains that he has been out of work for eight years. He has an excellent head for figures and is also very clever with his hands. But during his eight years on the dole he has received no advice about suitable work or been offered any employment. At thrity-two he was reduced to doing housework for his semi-invalid mother.

Government training centres for the disabled increased from thirteen in 1963 to forty-six in 1970. But as Mary Greaves of D.I.G. points out, rehabilitation for work is not enough on its own.

She says: 'Rehabilitation is composed of three parts –

medical, rehabilitation for living, and rehabilitation for work. There's a tendency to miss out the rehabilitation for living but if this is overlooked a person cannot cope with industrial rehabilitation. For instance, if a person cannot cope with getting out of bed and dressing he cannot go to work.

'It is also important for a person to have good appliances. If a disabled person is not comfortable with his appliances he cannot work well.'

Mary Greaves also holds strong views on the importance of a disabled person having some special skill or qualification to offer an employer. She speaks from experience:

'I had polio when I was three years old. When I left school no one thought of the possibility of my going to university. I learned shorthand and typing and for fourteen years I ran a commercial school and copying office from my own home. But I wasn't fulfilling myself. Then came the war in 1939 and I felt that with the shortage of labour my chance to obtain work in open employment had arrived. But I still couldn't get a job as a shorthand typist. It was then that I decided to improve my qualifications.'

After passing intermediate B.Sc. (Economics) she got a job as a statistician in the Ministry of Public Building and Works.

'I then went to the L.S.E. in the evenings to study for a degree in sociology. After that I attended Birkbeck College for a higher degree in industrial psychology. When I was fifty-seven I changed my job and went from the Ministry of Works to the National Economic Development Council.'

In her comfortable book-lined flat in central London, Mary Greaves sums up her experience from her wheelchair:

'It is terribly important for disabled people to get qualifications. I would not have got promotion without a degree. Disabled people should also go into growth industries where skills are scarce.'

But the winning of qualifications is sometimes only part of the battle. The case of Diana, a polio victim and psychology graduate in her early thirties, was reported by the *Sunday Times* in 1970. Although paralysed in both legs and one arm she could earn at least £30 a week in a full-time job with certain basic assistance, such as private accommodation, transport and home help. Instead she had lived in a hospital ward for five years and was restricted to doing a part-time job as a research assistant for which she earned about £5 a week.

Diana contracted polio when aged nineteen, shortly before she was due to go to university. She was still determined to have a worthwhile career and won a place at Bedford College in 1965 to study psychology. She had taught herself to breathe adequately when awake but required an iron lung at night. While a student she was housed at Western Hospital, Fulham, which had a respiratory unit. Soon after she graduated in 1968 the Western Hospital was closed and she was transferred to Stockwell. It took her over a year to find her research job. She then found an unfurnished house at Richmond, Surrey, with a rent of £8.50 a week. She arranged to let the first floor for £5. She asked Richmond Council to carry out necessary structural alterations on the ground floor – approximate cost £150 – and to provide a home help, cost £5 a week.

The hospital agreed to give her a respiratory machine on permanent loan and she applied to several charities for help with the running costs for the first year. But months passed and there was no action by the Richmond Council. It was reluctant to act until Diana had raised enough money to maintain herself for the first year. There was also a problem of transport to get her to and from work. But once she had got a full-time job she could probably have paid for that. The trouble was that without having the transport first she could not get such work.

The Richmond house stood empty meanwhile, the rent paid by a friend. Diana commented: 'I have done all in my power to improve my way of life but even after all this nothing is definite. It seems so wrong that I should be in hospital. Hospitals are for sick people. I am quite able to do a day's work.'

Lack of basic income – a small disability pension – to help a disabled person with accommodation and transport often prevents him from getting a job and achieving independence.

In March 1971 the Disablement Income Group published an important survey of the way in which seven European countries look after the financial needs of the handicapped. The report covered France, West Germany, the Netherlands, Denmark, Norway, Sweden and the U.K. It had this to say: 'Of the seven countries studied, Great Britain is the only one which does not have a disability pension as such for any category of disabled person other than the war and industrially disabled.'

The other six countries all award pensions to anyone whose disablement occurred during his working career. Denmark and Sweden go further than the rest by guaranteeing pensions for all disabled persons. The three Scandinavian countries also award pensions to disabled housewives.

* * *

Mr A. has cerebral palsy and because of his disability he earns much less than his ability justifies. He has a total income of £20 a week. Mrs A. was originally in normal health but now has a chronic psychiatric illness following a nervous break-down after the birth of her youngest child. She cannot leave her home alone and needs regular drug therapy. There are three children, all above average intelligence, but the two younger children have been seriously affected by the family problems. Mrs A. does not get exemption from prescription charges and they get no help towards a family car as psychiatric illness is not officially classified as a disability by the Government. Local social service work is not very good, but even if it were it would probably not be able to relieve the family of the continual strain of financial worry. They have tried to be independent, they have tried to save. They have only had two holidays in twenty-five years.

Chapter Five

A Home to Live In

A MARRIED couple with a disabled son aged twenty-four have been trying to get suitable accommodation for twelve years. Their son's wheelchair will not go through the doors to the toilet or bathroom. They write: 'Our son has to get as near as he can to the door and jump and catch hold of the door with his hands and drag his legs after him. Many is the time he has landed on the floor and as he cannot walk at all you will have some idea of the situation. He has to be carried up and down stairs. The last offer we had was a flat in a multi-storey block on the second floor which even the Welfare advised us not to take.'

* * *

An old age pensioner, totally blind in one eye and growing blind in the other is also disabled with arthritis in both legs and obliged to use a wheelchair. He is on the disabled register at the employment exchange. Yet he has been housed on the sixth floor of a multi-storey block. He has not been out of his flat for five years except for visits to the hospital for two operations. He has tried to get a flat on the ground floor 'so that I can belong to the human race again and be able to talk to people instead of being a prisoner in my own home just staring at the walls.'

* * *

Mrs White started labour while she was on her own in a room in South London and gave birth before the ambulance could be called. The child that was born suffered brain damage. Now seven years old the little boy, Peter, is totally dependent and mentally handicapped. He cannot do anything for himself. The family rented two rooms and a kitchen on the fourth floor of a tall terraced house in north London – but they shared the bathroom and toilet on the first floor. All went reasonably well until the second child was born and Peter became bigger and heavier so that his mother, a rather short woman, had great difficulty in carrying him up and down stairs. Life became increasingly difficult when Mrs White found herself pregnant again when the second child was only two years old. The local authority then offered the family accommodation on a modern housing estate. It was a flat on the fourth floor and was reached by lift. Mr White accepted because he feared he would not be offered anything else if he refused. There is a small entrance hall and two bedrooms at that level. The kitchen, living and bathrooms are reached by a steep staircase. The maisonette, in fact, is most unsuitable for a family with a severely handicapped child and two other young children. Peter has to remain in his bedroom when his father is out at work because his mother is unable to carry him up and down stairs. She is also unable to bath him or take him to the toilet without the help of the father. His food has to be taken down to his bedroom. Peter feels very isolated and alone downstairs while the rest of the family are in the living quarters above. Pram sheds are available for some maisonettes. The Whites were unable to obtain one, however, because 'the computer said so'. Their entrance hall is too small to store a wheelchair, pram and pushchair. A pram shed would have solved one of their problems, yet although most of the sheds were still not let, the authorities refused to allow them to have one.

*   *   *

Just before Christmas 1971, Derek Rowley, a forty-year-old unemployed kitchen worker, mentally retarded, was evicted from the council house in Stoke where he had lived all his life. The eviction took place despite an appeal from the local welfare services department that he should be permitted to stay on until more suitable accommodation could be found. He had lived alone in the house since his parents had died four years before. The local housing committee defended its action on the ground that the house was dirty and that there had been complaints from neighbours that it was used by homosexuals. Welfare workers who questioned Rowley were convinced that what the neighbours really saw was Rowley befriending other lonely men on the dole and inviting them home for a cup of tea.

* * *

A former miner, transformed into a chair-bound paraplegic by a pit accident six years before, had been re-housed from a colliery house into a council house on a new estate. The National Coal Board offered to share the cost of making any necessary alterations to the house to enable the man to cope. After many visits by council officials, many letters and much measuring, the man was informed that as it was a new estate plans could not be altered, and that in any case there were too many steps to build ramps over. The man has to manage with doors that are too narrow for his wheelchair and a toilet and bathroom at the top of a steep flight of stairs. His daughter writes: 'The situation is desperate and extremely disheartening for someone as active as my father . . .'

* * *

Nearly a quarter of Britain's housing – some four million dwellings – is officially unfit for habitation or lacks one or more of the basic amenities. Millions of people live in accommodation that lacks an indoor lavatory, fixed bath or piped hot water. Their rooms are damp, cramped and badly heated. It is wretched enough for anyone to live in such conditions in the 1970s. It is even worse for someone who is disabled. Yet because disabled people are often among the poorest in the land a high proportion of them are to be found buried away in squalid and depressing conditions. About a quarter of a million handicapped people are housed in slums. Moreover, for many of the disabled there is little or no escape from their decayed surroundings. Because of their disablement they are forced to spend virtually their whole time indoors. For them there is not even the break of eight or so hours a day in the relative cheer of a factory or office.

The worst housed are those disabled people who live virtually in one room with their families, sharing a tap and outside lavatory with several other families. Every drop of water required entails a climb up and down narrow, badly lit stairs to the communal tap. All hot water needed must be heated on the stove in the living-cum-bedroom which must act as bathroom, too. The best housed are those who live in specially designed bungalows or ground floor flats provided by themselves or more often by a local authority or charity. But only a few out of every hundred disabled people are so fortunate.

Between the worst and best stretches a wide range of housing, most of it in some way inadequate because of steps and stairs, narrow doorways and corridors, awkward heights of switches and plugs, cupboards and shelves, meters, sinks and taps. Stairs are the biggest problem. A large proportion of the disabled lack at least one of the basic amenities – a fixed bath, indoor lavatory or piped hot water. It does not require much imagination to appreciate the difficulties and embarrassments of a partly paralysed person confined to a wheelchair using an outdoor W.C. in wintry conditions.

The local authority has a key role to play in providing better accommodation for the disabled or making adaptations and improvements to their homes. Under the National Assistance Act 1948, town halls were empowered to make housing adaptations to make life easier for the handicapped. But that measure did not compel them to take action. The most common adaptations provided are ramps for steps, rails for baths and raised lavatory seats. People who are registered as disabled stand a better chance of getting such improvements carried out. But a lot of disabled people and their families simply do not know that local authorities are able to carry out such work free of charge. The provision of adaptations depends not only on the willingness of the authority to do the work but also on its enthusiasm in publicizing the service. Some authorities have been much better than others. Complaints about delay in making adaptations are legion. The experience of the Fishers is not uncommon . . .

Mrs Dorothy Fisher, a woman in her mid-fifties, has one leg amputated below the knee and also suffers from diabetes and arthritis. Her husband Fred, about ten years older, has muscular dystrophy and has not worked for over twenty years. In 1971, they were living in a Kensington council flat. Mrs Fisher realized after many attempts at using an artificial limb that she would never be able to manage one. Moreover, her arthritis made it impossible for her to use crutches and she could not operate a wheelchair in the flat because the doors were too narrow. So Mrs Fisher had to get about on her stump and her good knee. As for Mr Fisher, if he fell he was unable to pick himself up and had to wait to be lifted. The bedroom in the flat was so cold and damp that the couple moved their bed into the small living room. It was heated by a coal fire and the coal bunker was outside the front door. When coal had to be collected it was dragged by Mrs Fisher on her stump and good knee. The couple had complained that the flat was unsuitable when they were first put there by the council. They had been trying to leave for four years. For two or three years Guy's Hospital had been writing to the local authority urging that better accommodation should be provided. A number of newspapers also took up the case. Kensington claimed, however, that it had done its best to provide the Fishers with what they needed. The council had, in fact, made some minor adaptations including a rail in the bathroom and a rail and sloping curb outside the house. It argued, however, that it could not carry out major adaptations. And, having spent money on some improvements, it was reluctant to move the couple. Then early in 1971 Kensington at last decided that it could carry out some major adaptations such as widening doors and providing some easier form of heating. The council took this action only after the local M.P., Bruce Douglas-Mann, and a voluntary organization, citing the Morris Act, had taken up the case and local newspapers had given it publicity.

Complaints are not confined to the slowness of local officialdom. Some authorities cap sluggishness with unbelievable meanness. The head occupational therapist of a hospital management committee in Lancashire has told how it can take many months of nagging from himself and the consultant to persuade a local authority to provide aid which may cost very little. One patient was assessed one January for a raised lavatory seat at a cost of £2·50. After much nagging the local authority supplied this in the April – only to take it away again the following March in order to give it to an older person.

Some local authorities are so notoriously mean in their provision for the disabled that impaired people try not to move into their areas and as result their mobility is severely restricted. They and their families will turn down the chance of employment or promotion in such areas because of the lack of services. Yet as long ago as 1956 the Piercy Committee urged that all responsible for local authority housing schemes should bear in mind the needs of the disabled. The committee wanted accommodation to be designed without steps and with doors wide enough to allow the passage of wheelchairs.

The re-housing of disabled people in suitable accommodation has proved to be a particularly slow operation. A high proportion of those in bad housing have been on local authority waiting lists for several years. Moreover, there is strong evidence to suggest that such lists are far from complete. Reginald Freeson, who was Housing Parliamentary Secretary until Labour lost the 1970 General Election, revealed after losing office that while at his ministry he had made a broad calculation that housing lists in stress areas throughout the country reflected only about a quarter of the real need in the worst parts of Britain's cities. The figures had a special relevance to the chronically sick and disabled because they can be found in large numbers in such depressed areas.

When accommodation is eventually provided it is often in obviously unsuitable quarters, allocated by unthinking officials without regard to the needs of the people involved. A lot of disabled people become virtual prisoners in small flats perched high up in tall soulless blocks. They are cut off from their friends and relations, shops and entertainments.

Frank McElhone, Labour M.P. for Gorbals, Glasgow, has described what he and a team of volunteers found in a door-to-door survey in his constituency to track down handicapped people. 'Going round the houses from doorstep to doorstep I have found cases which would make one feel ill. There was one person who was incarcerated for three years in a flat in a multi-storey block. Getting that person a wheelchair in which to bring him back to civilization saved that man's mind. Some young people had the distressing experience of stopping an attempted suicide by a woman who was frustrated because of being incarcerated in her home twenty-four hours a day, seven days a week.'

It is not surprising that as disabled people become isolated they become paranoid, withdrawn and even suicidal. The need is not just for modern accommodation. It is certainly not for secluded accommodation cut off from social contact. Many people, in fact, even when they are short of basic amenities, refuse to be rehoused because they have got used to their surroundings and do not want to be cut off from friends and relations. This is particularly true of old people. The problem would be overcome if the authorities would rehouse people in their own localities. The biggest need, in fact, is for specially adapted houses within the community of which the disabled people are a part. If a disabled person is housed in such accommodation there is a good chance that he will not develop secondary psychiatric tendencies.

Some disabled people are able to build their own homes to suit their special needs. But even when they have the means they can encounter heartbreaking difficulties. Take this case from Oxfordshire:

Mrs H. applied for planning permission to build a bungalow for herself and three invalids. Every householder but one in her village supported them by signing a petition. But in spite of this the plans for the bungalow, which was to have special handrails and wide doors, were turned down. The house occupied by the family had three bedrooms upstairs but only one could be occupied – by Mrs H. herself.

Since her husband, a sufferer from rheumatoid arthritis, had fallen downstairs three times, and her invalid brother had fallen down twice, both men had slept downstairs. The bungalow was to be built on land belonging to the family and previously used for a garage. The Housing Ministry said that the local planning authority considered that there was genuine hardship involved but had finally decided that planning objections over-rode personal circumstances. Local authority representatives made the point that the invalids could perhaps be put in a home. The family, in despair, were willing to give an undertaking that the bungalow would be pulled down after their deaths. The Ministry dismissed their appeal.

*   *   *

The Multiple Sclerosis Society is one of a number of organizations for the handicapped taking special action to meet their housing needs. Since 1967 its policy has been to encourage the building of purpose-built housing near to a day-care centre. The Society, believing that the most desirable place for a disabled person to live is in his own home surrounded by his own family, is anxious to provide that set-up for as long as possible. If the housing is near a day-care centre the disabled person can be cared for there during the day, enabling the other partner to go out to work to support the family.

At the beginning of 1972 the Society was negotiating schemes in four areas – Bromley (40 to 48 flats), Liverpool (26 bungalows), Nottingham (6 houses, 6 bungalows) and Manchester.

The alternative to housing handicapped people in their own homes is to accommodate them in hospitals and community homes. The National Association for Mental Health has estimated that nearly half the mentally handicapped patients in England and Wales remain in hospital because they have nowhere else to go. A report by the Association in December 1971 stated that of 52,000 mentally handicapped patients 25,000 were ready to leave hospital. If adequate after-care treatment was available the problem of reintegrating such people into the community would be dramatically reduced. Recent surveys, such as one carried out at spinal units, have revealed in fact that badly disabled people living in their own homes – no matter how poor and inadequate – enjoy longer and happier lives than those living in institutions. Moreover, the effect on the family of a disabled person can be damaging when he is sent to a hospital or home. The break-up of family life can have serious effects on the children. The point has been made, for instance, that a high percentage of young men in borstal institutions come from families with disablement problems.

Such facts cast doubt on the wisdom of well intentioned policies as those of the Wilson Government in giving such high priority to the hospital building programme over the housing programme. Spending on hospital building under Labour increased by about fifty per cent, but its housing record was a bitter disappointment, particularly in the light of public pledges to achieve a target of 500,000 new dwellings a year. Ministers in the Labour Government were clearly influenced by advice from Whitehall that put emphasis on hospital rather than domiciliary care for the chronically sick and disabled. Former Minister David Ennals, who was Minister of State for Health in the Wilson Government, now concedes that such emphasis was wrong. He says: 'I am much more convinced than I was when in the Government of the need for community and domiciliary care,' and he talks about the 'essential importance of domiciliary services'. Ennals has been brought to that belief by his experience as campaign director for the National Association for Mental Health.

One recent survey has shown that some sixty per cent of the people in acute hospitals were not there because they were acutely ill. About fifteen per cent were there because they were unable to move around without assistance. But quite often such people could be discharged with safety if small adaptations, such as handrails in lavatories and bathrooms, were provided at home.

Apart from the general proposition that handicapped

people should, as far as possible, be cared for in their own homes there are special problems arising from the present haphazard system of treating such people in hospitals and institutions. A consultant psychiatrist writes: 'Working in a mental hospital perpetually reminds one of the harmful effect which admission to such an institution has on a patient's ability to cope with life in general. It is only too easy for a chronically sick person to be admitted to a mental hospital and then somehow to get stuck there and undergo a process of progressive institutionalization and delapidation. The majority of these patients do not really require hospitalization but are found in mental hospitals because there is nowhere else for them to go.'

An intelligent woman in her fifties wrote to Alfred Morris: 'I have been put in this geriatric hospital because I am suffering from a severe condition of rheumatoid arthritis. I am here with very old people, most of them quite oblivious to their surroundings. Because I am here I am being treated like an old woman before it is time for that. I am unhappy, desperate and in great distress. I have been shut up here for eighteen months and have never been so unhappy in all my life. For four and a half years I lived in a bedsitter flat where there was a warden. I had a setback with my arthritis and had to go to hospital for treatment. The warden wouldn't have me back in the home. She was afraid I was going to be a nuisance.'

Another woman wrote from Sheffield: 'I am not disabled, but because I have been beset with ill health for over twenty years I have been thrown into contact with the crippled and chronic sick. When someone falls victim of one of the terrible diseases such as multiple sclerosis or Parkinson's disease it is common practice to dump them in the geriatric wards of hospitals. Some are even put into asylums. I've seen poor souls with paralysed legs left lying or sitting for hours where they have fallen, having been brusquely told: 'You can stand up quite well if you really try.'

'Sick people, including myself, have been pushed out of doors in grinding cold weather and kept locked out in the courtyard for up to two hours although we had only just

enough strength to move at snail's pace. Among other forms
of treatment frequently employed is that of locking up a
person without access to any sanitary convenience and later
reviling her for "being dirty" if the demands of nature finally
overcome her willpower. There is also the forcible undressing
of a woman before a crowd of others while making vulgar
comments about any physical pecularities she may have . . . '

At a different level there is the problem of disabled people
who are left to rot in hospitals because of faulty diagnosis.
Baroness Masham told the House of Lords in May 1970 that
for the past nineteen months a man of twenty-nine, married
with two young children, had existed helpless in Middlesbrough General Hospital. When she visited him she discovered that he was a paraplegic, paralysed from the chest
down. 'He is riddled with pressure sores. His left leg is so
contracted that it cannot bend at the knee. His toes are like
fixed claws. Four months ago, having seen so many badly
injured people come in and walk out from his ward this man
contemplated taking his own life. After nineteen months in
hospital he has not started to be rehabilitated and his wife
has not even met the doctor in charge . . . In the same
ward is a man of thirty, also with a wife and two young
children. He is paralysed from the sixth and seventh cervical
vertebrae. After one week in hospital he was sat upright.
He turned blue and stopped breathing. He has been in the
hospital for nine weeks. These men have no feeling from
their injury down. They do not call out when their skin is
sore. Far more serious is the psychological pain. They lie
from day to day and worry about sex problems and how to
continue their lives. These were virile young men in the prime
of their lives. Before I left their wives begged me, with tears
in their eyes, to help get their husbands moved to a spinal
unit anywhere in the country. They asked me: are these places
only for people with money?'

Some of these paralysed spinal cases have been kept in
general hospitals, becoming increasingly crippled and depressed, although they have been only ten miles or so from a
spinal unit in which there were free beds.

If Britain's hospitals were not so full of people who are

not really sick enough to warrant hospitalization the over-worked staff would have more time to ensure that those really in need of medical attention received the appropriate treatment.

The growing use of 'day hospitals' for handicapped people is one way of emptying the beds in the wards and giving a new lease of life to men and women who would otherwise degenerate into institutionalized cabbages. For example, a woman in her mid-eighties who had part of her leg amputated and spent over three years in hospital has been enabled to live at home and do a lot for herself, thanks to such a day hospital. Elderly people attend as day patients and receive medical treatment, therapy, and entertainment in relaxed surroundings. One says: 'It is just like a club.' People can always be kept in overnight if necessary; the hospital medical staff can carry out their investigations while they are attending the patient.

The day hospitals not only cut the demand for beds in hospitals. They also reduce the demand for places in local authority welfare homes. The cost of day patients including transport is only about half the per-day cost of an in-patient, and as they attend only a few days a week their total cost is less than a quarter of that of the full-time in-patient. More-over, after a month or so of medical treatment and occu-pational therapy they can often dispense with regular hospital treatment altogether.

Chapter Six

Getting Around

A DISABLED man was driving a Government issued three-wheeled invalid car in blustery weather. The unstable light-weight little vehicle rocked in alarming fashion – as it usually did in bad conditions. Suddenly it was caught by a particularly strong gust of wind. The next thing the driver knew was that he and the car were upside down in a ditch. As he was paralysed from the waist down he could not get out of the upturned vehicle. He was trapped in it for fourteen hours. No one saw him until the following morning when a passer-by noticed the upturned wheels beneath the hedgerow. The driver was rescued, shaken but smiling. If he had been a haemophiliac, prone to internal bleeding when jolted, he might well have died.

* * *

Mr A. is paralysed in all four limbs as a result of contracting polio at the age of fourteen. He has to be washed, dressed and helped to the lavatory. But he recently got his first job in an office because he is able to use an electric typewriter, telephone and dictaphone with the aid of POSSUM* apparatus. Soon after starting work, however, he discovered that he would not be able to continue without his own transport. He and his fiancée – now his wife – managed to buy a car. His wife takes him to and from work as well as doing a full-time job herself. If she was not working they could not meet

---

* (for description of POSSUM see chapter The Life Machines.)

the loan charges, repayments and cost of running the car. They receive no help from the authorities, although if Mr A. had been less severely disabled he would have been eligible for a Government one-seat, three-wheeler invalid car to drive himself. Yet without his present car Mr A. could not work. And without a job he would be dependent on the State.

* * *

A middle-aged man suffering from spina bifida and using crutches and surgical supports saved enough to buy a mini car. But, as so often happens with disabled people, he lost his job and had to sell the car. As his wife suffered from diabetes, he applied for a State mini car. Instead he was issued with a one-seat three-wheeler – for his personal use only. They were a devoted couple, always in each other's company and their main pleasure was visiting a wide circle of friends. But now when they went visiting he went by tri-car while his wife went by public transport. They were robbed of much of the pleasure of their outings. Moreover, the arrangement was complicated by the need for the wife to have injections of insulin three times a day.

On one occasion they set out to visit parents sixteen miles away. The husband waited at the bus stop to see his wife safely aboard. As they waited together, however, she became faint and confused due to her illness. He told her to sit beside him in the little car while he gave her sugar and as they sat there, the bus went passed the stop. In desperation he decided to carry her as a passenger, although he knew it was against the law. Within half a mile of their destination they were stopped by a police car. The woman was ordered from the car and had to walk the remainder of the journey. The man received a reprimand and warning'

After this embarrassing and heartbreaking experience their visits to friends became fewer. But if the man went out alone in the tri-car his wife worried in case it broke down. Her health began to break down and aggravated her diabetes. She was admitted to hospital. Soon after returning home she suffered a mental breakdown. Her doctors say she should not go out alone on public transport.

Michael Flanders, entertainer, speaking from personal experience as a disabled person, has said: 'Given enough slaves, very few places are totally inaccessible to the disabled but it would be a help if the people and bodies concerned could take steps to make life easier for us or preferably remove them.'

* * *

Much of the public transport system could have been designed by a sadistic physical training instructor previously employed on devising assault courses for commandos. Travelling on public transport, especially at rush hours, is often a trying and tiring experience for the able-bodied. For disabled people it can be a nightmare. Many of them find travel by public transport the most worrying and difficult part of trying to live normal lives. They will turn down social engagements and even jobs because they cannot face it. Much of the system, in fact, requires that people should be not only fit but agile. Take buses: the ordeal often begins with a long wait in a queue exposed to all weathers, followed by a scramble to board the vehicle when it at last arrives. Passengers are faced with high steps to board the bus, narrow gangways, narrow seats and little or no room for stowing equipment. If the lower deck is full, steep, narrow stairs with an awkward bend have to be negotiated to reach the upper deck – usually while the bus is lurching on its way. Drivers and conductors seem so hard pressed for time that they rarely give passengers time to take their seats before the vehicle is moving.

Tube trains present special problems of access – by escalators or deep stairs. Main line trains face the traveller with high boarding steps and a dangerous gap between platform and carriage; narrow corridors and – in modern trains – narrow seating in an open-plan arrangement, small luggage racks and narrow doors.

Faced with such a system it is not surprising that many disabled people opt out and decide to stay at home. They remain cut off from social contact, from shops, from employment and from holidays. The alternative is to have some private means of transport. But as most disabled people are already hard-up the purchase of a car is usually beyond them. If they are badly disabled they are, in any case, incapable of driving. A person suffering from a wasting disease can, in fact, find himself transformed gradually over the years from someone able to tackle the public transport assault course or drive his own car, to a disabled driver travelling alone in a Government-provided invalid tri-car until eventually he becomes incapable of driving and is reduced to the role of a disabled passenger isolated at home and receiving no Government assistance.

The British Government for some years has recognized the importance of mobility for the disabled. It has taken some steps to help. Yet its policy is criticised for anomalies and shortcomings. That policy has been explained at various times in these words: 'The arrangements for providing powered vehicles for disabled persons – or for giving some assistance in lieu – all depend on the disabled person being able to drive the vehicle. The concept is that of restoring to an individual as much personal physical mobility as it is possible to provide . . . The National Health Service three-wheeler is in our view basically a kind of artificial limb.'

The Government provides the single-seater invalid tricycle for people in several categories. It is maintained and insured free of cost and an allowance of £5 a year was made towards the cost of petrol until February 1972. The alternative of a small, four-seater car has been available for some years to war pensioners; to two members of the same family who are both entitled to an invalid tricycle; and to a husband and wife when one is eligible and the other is blind. Certain categories of handicapped people can also recover the cost of converting the controls of a private car once every five years up to a maximum of £90.

The Government applies no means test for this assistance but equally takes no heed of any extra financial problem faced by some disabled people. There are other disadvantages built into the system. The invalid tricycle, for instance, is a single-seat vehicle. The disabled driver is not allowed to carry a passenger. No account is taken of the family responsibilities or social needs of the disabled in this respect. The policy is also based on the *ability* to drive – rather than a disability. The disabled driver is in most cases forced to drive alone – husband separated from wife, disabled mother from her children. But the needs of the disabled passenger have been largely ignored. In fact, once a person has become so disabled that he cannot drive he is left with next to no Government assistance for road travel. The more disabled you are and the more help you need, the less you receive.

A disabled passenger explains: 'I have been polio-disabled since the age of eighteen and am now thirty-one. I am confined to a wheelchair and have movement only in my left forearm, wrist and hand. Although I qualify for an invalid carriage my disability is severe enough to prevent my being able to drive one. I am a writer and find it necessary for my work to go out and meet people and experience the outside world. Eighteen months ago I got married and, as we cannot afford a car, I relied on my wife pushing me for outdoor excursions. Six months ago we had a baby. Obviously my wife cannot push both me and the child; equally obviously we cannot leave the baby alone in the house . . . ' Not until February 1972, were disabled mothers with young children allowed a normal car. An example of their problems is this letter: 'My wife is disabled as a result of polio some twelve years ago. She has a Ministry invalid tricycle which is of great assistance to her but it has one very serious drawback in that she is unable to carry passengers. We have two young boys aged five and seven years who have to be taken to and collected from school each day. I am a police officer on shift duties and more often than not I am not available to take or collect the boys. My wife has to rely very much on assistance from other mothers which, although very willingly given, is a constant worry to her. As I am on duty most weekends, further difficulties arise if she wishes to take the children out.'

Baroness Masham, herself disabled and speaking from a wheelchair, told the House of Lords in one debate: 'I am the mother of an adopted daughter aged five. She is very pretty with blonde hair and blue eyes. I live three-quarters of a mile from the nearest primary school. I know that it would be impossible for me to allow her to walk to school. With so many sex maniacs around no mother could rest until she knew her daughter was safely home. Think what terrible frustration the mother must suffer who cannot take her daughter to school.'

A disabled mother of two girls wrote to the Central Council for the Disabled: 'I encountered a most terrible and distressing problem when my eldest child became old enough to go to school. I found that the Education Department could do nothing to help me get my little girl from our bungalow to her school. The Education Department sent me to the Health Department who said they had no means of helping me and referred me back to the Education Department. I was told that no help could be given towards the cost of a taxi service and that no passenger could be carried in my invalid tricar. The Welfare Officer promised to contact some mothers whose children would be starting school to see if they could accompany my daughter. Three days before my daughter was due to start I received a letter from the Welfare Officer with the names and addresses of two women asking me to contact them as she had not had time to do so. In the event my daughter started school accompanied by a lady who passed our door but after a month she decided to get a job so that arrangement finished. For a week or so my five-year-old wandered home alone but it reduced her to tears. I blew up the education officer on the phone and told him she wouldn't be able to go to school any more. I rang up my M.P. who came to see me and strangely enough after this the authorities arranged an escort to school and there was no more trouble. A year later when my younger girl needed the company of a nursery school it all began again . . .'

The husband of a woman suffering from multiple sclerosis applied for an invalid carriage for her but was told her disability was too serious for her to have one. The alternative in order to ensure that she got out was for him to buy a car. He was advised by his local tax office: 'There must be many disabled people in this situation – too incapacitated to manage an invalid car but unable to get any relief towards the expenses of running and maintaining a car by the family.'

A woman writes from Leicestershire: 'My husband has

an invalid car but my son and I cannot travel with him and this is a great worry. We cannot afford a family car as the savings we had were used up when my husband could not obtain employment. When repairs have to be done to the car it is a matter or waiting two weeks – even for a new tyre. During this period we have to hire a taxi to get my husband to work – or rely on the neighbours who are not really very sympathetic.'

Mr John Cordle, Conservative M.P. for Bournemouth East, told the Commons in May 1971 of a young man in his constituency virtually housebound and deprived of any pleasure as a result of an accident in 1968. He had become a severe paraplegic. His wife was aged twenty-two and he had two small daughters. A social worker had reported that on one or two occasions it had been hoped to arrange transport for him to attend a day centre but unfortunately he had become ill and it had not been possible to do it. He had been assessed for an invalid tricar but had turned this down partly because of his wish to have a specially adapted Ministry car in which to take his family out, and partly because he felt an invalid car would draw attention to his disabilities. The social worker commented: 'There is a tendency to treat a disabled person and his family as separate entities and in this particular case I feel it is essential to consider them as a family unit. The eldest child, already attending school, is an intelligent little girl but far too solemn and quiet for her age and in all probability this is partly due to the fact that due to lack of transport she is precluded from simple family pleasures such as going to the beach, into the country or to the shops . . . '

The invalid tricar not only isolates the disabled driver. It can let him down badly. It has a reputation for frequent breakdowns and bad road-holding. An experienced driver reports that he has been spun round completely in a circle on a tar macadam road in summer when hit by a cross wind from a side street. A sixty-one-year-old disabled housewife, married to a disabled man, says of her tricycle: 'It is very unreliable. I never know when I set off if it will break down somewhere and that I will be taken home by some kind person while the car is taken to the authorized repairers. This has happened so many times I have lost count.'

Graham Hill, the world champion racing driver, drove a three-wheeler when disabled in a driving accident. He said afterwards that, in racing parlance, he felt like a mobile chicane with traffic trying to dodge round the outside of him and he unable to keep up. Hill has argued that a three-wheeler with a wheel in the front is the most dangerous form of tricycle because such a car, when moving at any speed going round a corner will tend to roll and throw all the weight on a part of the vehicle where there is no wheel. He went to discuss the problem with Lord Crawshaw at the House of Lords before a crucial debate and commented: 'Surely to goodness we can approach some of the large motor companies about producing a suitable vehicle. What is wanted is a four-wheeled vehicle with at least two seats, mass produced by a company such as the British Motor Corporation, or Ford. Hill took the matter up with Lord Stokes, chairman of B.M.C., who said he was anxious to co-operate.

Baroness Masham has described how before she was married she used to drive a ministry three-wheeler. 'This vehicle proved so unreliable that every time I went out I took a long rope so that when I broke down I could be towed to the nearest garage. Most garages didn't know how to mend it and they wasted hours of time trying to find out. I do not think this is a suitable vehicle for the sufferers from severe haemophilia . . . '

It is not just that sufferers from internal bleeding could die if such a vehicle were to overturn in a ditch. There is the bigger problem that arises from the fact that a sudden twist or jolt can bring on an internal haemorrhage. They therefore require a vehicle that will give them a smooth ride and one in which they can carry a passenger in case of emergency. The Government at last accepted this point in February, 1972, and announced that people suffering from haemophilia could have a four-wheeled car instead.

Despite mounting complaints and evidence Governments have continued to argue that the invalid tricycle is a reliable vehicle. But basically Whitehall has opposed the general introduction of a four-wheeled vehicle on grounds of cost. This extra cost, however, would arise not so much from the higher price of a four-wheeled compared to a three-wheeled vehicle. It arises from the more telling fact that the demand for a four-wheeler – so much safer and more useful – would be very much greater. The government, on grounds of economy, has preferred to provide a vehicle that it knows is unacceptable to a large number of people who need a car. This policy has been supported by both Labour and Tory administrations.

Disabled drivers and those driving them have also encountered great problems with parking. Baroness Masham has described how, on one occasion, a young policeman pounced on her after she had driven around Harrogate about six times. She was trying to collect a parcel from a shop. To encourage him to be helpful she explained that she had a special yellow badge issued to help disabled people get parking space. But he retorted after inspecting it.: 'That was issued in the North Riding. Harrogate is in the West Riding.'

The policeman's attitude is apparently not untypical according to reports from other disabled people. And drivers of disabled passengers waiting for them to finish their business in a shop or office have all too often been moved along by unsympathetic traffic wardens. Sometimes such officials are deliberately using their powers in a heartless manner but sometimes the trouble has arisen from ignorance. A very badly disabled woman was taken shopping by her husband who parked six inches outside the parking line to get the wheelchair out of the boot. When they returned they found a ticket from the police telling them to report to the police station. There they had to wait while the officer concerned finished his tea. But when the husband explained what had happened the policeman replied: 'How was I to know? You had no sign to show me that you had a disabled passenger.'

Faced with so many problems and slow-moving Governments content to perpetuate anomalies in the interests of economy – often false economy – the disabled drivers have organized themselves for action. The Invalid Tricycle

Association was formed in 1948 and changed its name later
to the Disabled Drivers' Association. It has about 6,000
members who pay a subscription of £1 a year. Charles
Pocock, the present general secretary, was appointed in 1963.
Energetic, articulate and practical he works from an office
in his bungalow at Wickford, Essex. He is also national
chairman of the Association for Research into Restricted
Growth. His own height is 4 ft. 1 in.

Charles Pocock's Disabled Drivers' Association is a
pressure group to be reckoned with, especially when assisted
at the Commons by back-benchers of the calibre of Neil
Marten, Tory M.P. for Banbury. At the end of 1971 they had
reached an important stage in their campaigning. Up to then
they had never met the head of a Whitehall department and
had been obliged to deal with junior ministers, but on 7
December, with Alfred Morris and James Loring, Director
of the Spastics Society, they went to Downing Street for
discussions with Edward Heath, the Prime Minister. Pocock
said later: 'He didn't brush us aside. He encouraged discussion. I think he gave us a very sympathetic hearing.'

Pocock believes the Association's biggest achievement is
the recognition by the public that mobility is not an end in
itself but 'a key that invariably opens the door of opportunity'. He says: 'What can you think of that doesn't involve
mobility. The invalid trike, although it introduced mobility
and provided employment opportunities created other problems. The trike savours of the old philosophy that it is good
enough to pat the disabled person on the head and give him
a couple of bob. You can't take the disabled person and deal
with him in isolation. He is set in a family, a community,
a society. Consequently when you provide a service for him
you have to see the totality of his need. We are now getting
that message through.

'We don't say that society owes disabled people a living.
But it should remove the obstacles relating to mobility,
appliances and finance; and, having removed them, it should
provide opportunities.'

But he concedes that not all disabled people agree with
that assessment. There is a sense in which he believes the

disablement problem is not unlike the colour problem. Some disabled people, like some coloured people, want preferential treatment. They are not always the most deserving.

The Association achieved a major breakthrough in February, 1972. Sir Keith Joseph, Secretary of State for Social Services, announced a package of measures, including the introduction of an allowance of £100 a year to enable disabled drivers to forgo the three wheeler, and run a vehicle of their own choice.

The Association is now campaigning for the appointment of a special Minister for the Disabled. Pocock explains: 'At present we have to deal with about half-a-dozen different departments.'

A determined campaign to improve all forms of transport for handicapped people is being conducted by the Joint Committee on Mobility for the Disabled under the vigorous chairmanship of Peter Large, himself severely disabled. They have pointed out that suggestions for making public transport usable by the disabled are usually countered by the argument that there are too few to warrant the expense of adapting buses and trains. Yet there is growing evidence that transport systems unsuitable for the disabled are unsuitable for many others, too. Moreover, it is argued that the total number of 'disabled' travellers is sufficiently great to justify a careful reappraisal of transport systems. The temporarily disabled, for instance, include pregnant women and people who may have strained a wrist or broken a limb.

In October, 1971, however, Mr Large's committee complained strongly that no progress was being made. Indeed, new transport systems were even less accessible to disabled travellers than older systems. They pointed out: 'No progress is being made because there is no policy covering these problems of the disabled traveller, and there is no policy because the total problem and its possible solution have not yet been investigated. It may be that there are few disabled people travelling because some cannot use existing systems and others are discouraged from using them because they are so inconvenient.'

Lord Wynne-Jones, who has artificial hips, has told the House of Lords about his travel problems: 'One of the enormous difficulties with which any person who is arthritic is faced, is getting in and out of public service vehicles and in getting any type of help.'

Lord Crawshaw, who uses a wheelchair, has described how he always travels in the guard's van on trains: 'On a mild day that is all right. . . I travel with everything from motor bikes to mail bags and maggots . . . '

The failure of the authorities to make proper provision for disabled travellers means that they must suffer much discomfort and indignity – or stay at home.

Every month a group of helpless cripples are loaded into a furniture van in one town to be taken from their homes to a tea and concert organized by the local Cripples Guild. They are strapped to the sides of the gloomy vehicle to prevent their chairs sliding about. There is no light and there are no windows to look from. They are obliged to put up with these conditions because the local authority has failed to make an ambulance available.

~~~~~~

Chapter Seven

The Life Machines

FOR MORE than a year after she contracted polio Barbara Pitchford just lay in bed and stared at the ceiling. Five years later she was described by Wendy Hughes of the *Sunday Times* as 'an ordinary middle-class housewife'. Her life had begun again in November 1966 when the British Polio Fellowship had supplied her with a POSSUM machine. POSSUM is short for Patient Operated Selector Mechanism. In Latin, *possum* means 'I can' or 'I am able'.

With a slight movement of the toes of her right foot Mrs Pitchford can operate switches on her POSSUM unit controlling radio, television, heat, light, telephone, electric blanket, bell to ring for assistance, and the apparatus that enables her to read micro-filmed books. With the aid of POSSUM she oversees the running of her modern home in Sussex and also works as a part-time typist from her sitting-room. Mrs Pitchford explains that it gives her a feeling of independence and achievement when she has done a day's work. How much better than feeling bored and frustrated.

*   *   *

Hilary Pole became crippled when she was twenty-one. That was over twelve years ago. She cannot speak, can only breathe through a specially developed ventilator, she has to be fed and cannot keep her eyes open. The only muscles in her body capable of movement are those in her big toes. She is, in fact, one of the most seriously disabled people in Britain.

Yet Hilary, of Walsall, Staffordshire, has a lively brain, great courage and enormous determination. She also has POSSUM. And thanks to her own qualities and this remarkable machine, she manages to enjoy life. POSSUM helps her to control about a dozen electrical devices, including a typewriter. She composes poems. Here is one of them:

> I have a world that's
> 　　mine alone,
> A world where no one
> 　　else can roam . . .
> Of roads I've walked
> And hills I've climbed
> Woods and fields
> 　　stored in mind.
> So if at night I cannot
> 　　sleep
> I do not end up
> 　　counting sheep.
> Instead,
> I think of days gone by,
> Of picnics 'neath a clear
> 　　blue sky.

Her mother has said: 'Hilary is living more fully than many people with all their faculties.'

Through her POSSUM Hilary has explained what it means to her: 'It is really part of me. It is my independence and enables me to have a private life.'

*　　*　　*

Mrs Daphne Whitehead of Cheltenham, suffering from the after effects of respiratory polio, has limited movement in her left arm and hand. At one time her only two aids, apart from a telephone, were a piece of string which operated her light and a bell which rang upstairs in her housekeeper's flat. She has said: 'I was also given a potato holder, but what I was supposed to do with it I cannot imagine.' We called this the 'string era'. But now a special panel of microswitches with finger-tip control has been designed to enable her to operate a control system called PILOT (Patient Initiated Light Operated Tele-Control). With that amazing equipment she can now independently operate the T.V., light and fire. She can also lower and raise the bed, answer the front door through a speaker and let in visitors, and ring a bell in the upstairs flat when she needs the housekeeper. Mrs Whitehead has said: 'How I ever managed before I don't know, as this equipment really transformed my domestic life. My only complaint is that I have to do everything around here these days.'

*　　*　　*

The time has passed when to be severely disabled meant that a person became a virtual cabbage – a helpless wreck dependent entirely on their family or the State.

The truth – astonishing as it may seem to many – is that even men and women almost totally paralysed can today live at home with their families, continue their education and help to support themselves with work of use to the community. Modern technology is responsible for this miracle. It has produced a wide range of electronic aids, of which the POSSUM equipment is the finest example, to enable people who are severely disabled to exercise control over equipment necessary to run a home or a business. By blowing into a tube, or by the flicker of a toe or a finger on a microswitch, the disabled person can control such equipment as radio, television, heat, light, telephone, door, electric typewriter, tape recorder and calculating machine. The POSSUM, the most advanced equipment of its kind in the world, was invented by Reginald Maling, who conceived the idea in 1960 when visiting a paralysed friend in hospital. The patient was able to summon assistance by blowing a whistle hanging from the ceiling and Maling decided that this ability to blow could be used to operate machinery. POSSUM was developed with the aid of the Polio Research Fund and has been available under the National Health Service – free of charge – since 1966.

Yet, despite the obvious value of such equipment and its

availability, only just over two hundred POSSUM units had been supplied to disabled people up to the end of 1971. The Health Department had informed all National Health doctors and hospitals, but many local authorities had done nothing to publicize the service and many doctors appear to have ignored the circular about the new equipment.

Lewis Carter-Jones, Labour M.P. for Eccles, who has been a tireless and vigorous campaigner for better equipment for the handicapped, complained strongly in Parliament in 1971 about the failure to make it generally known that such useful equipment as POSSUM was available to those in need. He pointed out that a person's chances of getting such equipment depended very much upon where he lived. In London, for instance, the disabled living in the South West Metropolitan area have a four times better chance of getting advanced technological help than those living in the North West area. In the whole of East Anglia, an area covering some two million people, only one POSSUM had been prescribed. In Glasgow there was not even one.

The equipment is not cheap. A POSSUM machine can cost between £300 and £600. But the saving to the tax-payer far outweighs that expense. This is because it costs over £100 a week to keep a patient in a hospital intensive care unit, whereas if POSSUM is supplied patients can often be discharged to their homes. If Whitehall and local authorities carried out proper cost-benefit analysis it is clear from such figures as those just quoted that government would discover that the real cost of providing the best possible equipment and care for the disabled is much less than officials have ignorantly advised. In the absence of such analysis, however, the authorities are haunted by false fears of the cost of providing services and fail to make information available to the public. When this is coupled with what amounts to criminal neglect by some officials and doctors in failing to act on circulars, there emerges an appalling picture of wasted opportunity.

Mr Marsh Dickson, President of the National Campaign for the Young Chronic Sick, has described his own family's experience in recent years of the failure of local authorities to provide information about equipment. His wife Dorothy, suffering from multiple sclerosis and unable to read, write, stand or feed herself, was entitled to a POSSUM. Her general practitioner was asked to arrange a visit to the consultant at the Middlesex Hospital. But the hospital was most discouraging and said that to the best of its knowledge people with Mrs Dickson's disease were not entitled to such equipment. Fortunately, however, Mr Dickson knew this was not true and fought on. Eventually, long after the average person would have given up, he gained the support of the consultant and obtained the POSSUM. At that time there were three POSSUMS in use in the wealthy boroughs of Kensington and Chelsea – and in each case the information about them had come not from a hospital or from the local authority but from voluntary organizations.

Carter-Jones, who has also spent a lot of time on research into the economics of disability, claims that in all the work he has done on the subject he has never come across a case in which the State has been worse off economically by giving help.

There is the case of Paul Bates, for instance, who got polio in Malaya in 1954 and became known as the horizontal man because he was permanently on his back. He was even unable to breathe without a respirator. But Bates was provided with POSSUM equipment and with its assistance was soon earning enough to qualify for paying income tax. If he had been dependent on the State he would have cost taxpayers at least £100 a week in an intensive care unit.

Disabled people do not always need equipment as sophisticated as POSSUM to enable them to earn a living. A typical case dealt with by Carter-Jones concerns a man, Harry Evans, who went to his 'surgery' suffering from a severe spinal complaint. He was terribly worried because he was dependent on his wife. He was drawing only £5 18s. a week from the State and had to rely on his apprentice son giving him a packet of cigarettes from time to time. Such an existence made Mr Evans – a skilled draughtsman – feel extremely depressed. He could have carried on work as a draughtsman at home, but his problem was one of communication. He needed a

telephone so that he could get in touch with potential employers and they could get in touch with him. On his income
of under £6 a week he simply could not afford one. Finally
an approach was made to the Department of Employment
and they provided a phone. Not long after that Harry Evans
was able to tell his doctor: 'I don't want a medical certificate
thank you very much. I'm now paying income tax on the
earnings I've got by being given a telephone.'

*   *   *

Many people suffering from kidney disease have died
unnecessarily in recent years due to the failure of the authorities to adapt their homes to enable them to take artificial
kidney machines. The equipment, called a dialysis machine,
cleans the patient's blood, and enables him to lead something
like a normal life. Normal, that is, except that the patient
has to spend thirty hours a week linked up to the machine.
A patient first receives treatment on a kidney machine at a
hospital, but places are severely limited and he must eventually go on to home dialysis or receive a kidney transplant.
One of the most advanced units in the country is at Cardiff
Royal Infirmary where twelve machines were treating thirty
people a week at the end of 1971. It is supported financially
by the Kidney Research Unit for Wales Foundation, a highly
successful money-raising charity. Ideally each patient should
have three ten-hour sessions a week on the machine, but
because of the problem of travelling long distances to and
from the infirmary some patients were having two spells
of about fourteen hours each.

In June 1971, a startling medical report alleged that more
than eighteen kidney patients had died between 1967-70,
mostly in the London area, because of red tape and delay
by local authorities in adapting houses to take kidney machines. The charges were made in a report by Dr Peter
Gower, of Charing Cross Hospital Medical School at
Fulham Hospital, and social worker Mrs Richenda Stubbs.
The allegations arose from a survey of thirty-five kidney
failure patients from one London hospital. The report
complained that hospital beds were blocked for dying

patients because of administrative delays by the Greater London Council and other local authorities. The homes of kidney patients could be converted to take dialysis machines in two or three months, but inquiries had revealed that there had been a total of seventy-two months, unnecessary delay in adapting the homes of thirty-five people who had died. The report argued that even if it were conceded that only half the total of deaths in the three-year study were due directly to delays this meant that eighteen patients had lost their lives from that cause.

Once a patient has a machine at home and can have three spells on it a week he feels a big improvement. Not having to travel to hospital and spend so much time there also makes it easier for a kidney patient to keep a job. Mr X. was travelling sixty miles to Cardiff twice a week for treatment and had not worked for three years. He would leave home at 8 a.m. on Tuesday and get home at noon on Wednesday. He explained: 'What firm would employ a man under those circumstances?'

By providing equipment to enable severely disabled people to do things for themselves the authorities are not only giving a new lease of life to the handicapped, they are also liberating those members of the family who would otherwise have been tied down to the job of caring for their every need. This is another important factor often overlooked by those assessing the cost of helping the disabled.

One of the big needs now is for cheaper types of control equipment that could be used by elderly disabled people to enable them to live at home, instead of having to be put into hospitals and institutions.

One organization working with great effect to improve the equipment available for the handicapped is the Disabled Living Foundation. The symbol of this independent charitable body is a little house with two disabled occupants, one on crutches and able to walk, the other confined to a wheelchair. The middle of the house containing the disabled people has dovetails around it, and with the help of those dovetails the disabled people fit snugly into their environment.

The chairman of the Foundation is Lady Hamilton, wife of

Sir Patrick Hamilton, who has applied her considerable energy, intelligence and organizing ability to the task of tackling the problems of daily living that confront all types of disabled people. She explains that the object of the foundation is to study the life environment of the disabled – their whole life from the onset of disability to death.

She stresses: 'We differ from ordinary research study organizations in that our research is a preliminary to doing something about it. If you do research and do nothing about it or get no one else to do anything you might just as well not have done it in the first place. Very often we are pioneering – sometimes world pioneering. There is very little written material existing and this leads to two consequences: a lack of training material for people professionally concerned; and a lack of generally accepted standards of good practice.'

Up to 1970 Lady Hamilton and her associates operated as the Disabled Living Activities Group of the Central Council for the Disabled. They broke away, however, because the Central Council was concerned principally with the physically handicapped, whereas they were anxious to work on behalf of people suffering from all forms of disability, including mental trouble. In January 1970, with a grant of £50,000 from a private trust, the Foundation set up a remarkable Aids Centre in Kensington High Street, London, for the display of a wide range of equipment for the disabled. The centre is designed to inform people working in the field, such as social workers, hospital staff and local government officials. In 1971 it was visited both by Prime Minister Edward Heath and the Secretary of State for Health and Social Security, Sir Keith Joseph. The exhibits range from simple, specially designed clothing to highly sophisticated POSSUM equipment. There are electrically controlled beds that can stand or sit a person up and lie him down; ripple mattresses which ensure that a disabled person is never lying on the same pressure area for more than ten minutes, thus preventing painful pressure sores; many varieties of chairs including some electric types that can be operated by sucking or blowing down a tube; hoists and slings for moving people from bed to chair or chair to bath; and so on . . .

A panel of experts has been assembled to advise on the design of equipment under the chairmanship of Lady Hamilton. She believes that in a period when money is short the government should employ its limited resources on research. If and when finance became more plentiful Whitehall would then be ready to undertake the production of new lines in the knowledge that they were the best possible designs. At the end of 1971 the Foundation was embarking on action to improve existing aids. It began with hoists as there had been a lot of complaints about them. The Foundation always has a disabled person on its advisory panels and their advice on practical problems is, of course, invaluable. In a lot of fields the people concerned do not know what type of equipment to provide. In the housing field, for instance, there is the simple example of door handles. If you are a disabled person with impaired hands you have great difficulty in using doors because you cannot grip the handles. The Foundation did some research on this and discovered that there is one type of handle which disabled people can manage. It would be of great help if that type of handle were now to be fitted to all doors in premises used by the impaired and elderly.

Important work on equipment is being sponsored by the National Fund for Research into Crippling Diseases. This organization, better known to the public by its more emotive slogan of Action for the Crippled Child, devotes about a tenth of its effort to the equipment problem. Sadly, due to past differences of opinion, the National Fund was having very little to do with the Disabled Living Foundation at the beginning of 1972. Duncan Guthrie, Director of the National Fund, is a remarkable man. Like Lady Hamilton of the Disabled Living Foundation, he is a strong personality. He started the organization in 1952 with virtually no money, after working on the Festival of Britain for the Arts Council. His eldest daughter had contracted poliomyelitis in 1949 at the age of eighteen months. His experience of her illness made it clear that the medical profession knew very little about polio and he decided to set up an organization to finance research into that then all too prevalent disease. He is a bulky, bearded man with a touch of the impressario and a background ranging from banking to acting plus an impressive war record, much of it spent behind German and Japanese lines.

Guthrie is also Director of the Central Council for the Disabled, a voluntary body which, like so many others, was set up in 1919 at the end of the First World War. He took on this job in the late 1960s as part of an operation to reduce the number of organizations working in the field, and so cut the administration costs. As a result of his dual role the National Fund and the Central Council had, in fact, started to work quite closely together by the beginning of 1972. Leading personalities in some other organizations, however, were looking less kindly on the idea of mergers.

The National Fund has a committee on research on apparatus for the disabled. It has given grants to a number of organizations including the Research Institute for Consumer Affairs, for work on evaluating specially designed aids and normal domestic equipment for use by disabled people; and the North Staffordshire Medical Institute for research into the use of plastics in the production of aids and appliances.

At his National Fund office in Vincent Square, London, Guthrie says of the future: 'I'd like a better wheelchair – or some other equipment to get people around. I think perhaps some kind of Hovercraft is the answer. The disabled person could perhaps sit in a type of bicycle saddle that would bring him up to the same height as people walking with him. Disabled people often feel most cut off when being wheeled in chairs because the friends with them talk over their heads.'

He is anxious to get away from the purely philanthropic 'trips to the seaside' approach to work for the handicapped; he tells voluntary bodies that the most useful work they can do is to persuade local technical colleges to think about designing better equipment.

The National Fund receives no help from the government, which spends much less than £½ million a year on research for the disabled. The budget for research and development projects for the defence programme in 1971 was £259 million. It was increased by £66 million in 1972.

The heartbreaking problem of trying to get financial support for the production of equipment is highlighted by the experience of John Collins, inventor of PILOT.

John Collins invented PILOT after Ann Armstrong, the disabled editor of *Responaut*, a remarkable magazine provided by and for people aided by respirators and other gadgets, explained that she wanted a piece of equipment to help her to type more easily. She had POSSUM but it did not suit her purpose because it was necessary to learn a code. She wanted to deal in letters and words rather than operate a machine by sucking and blowing. Collins – chief research engineer for Hugh Steeper Ltd, makers of artificial limbs and other rehabilitation equipment – set to work to design a light-operated typewriter.

But when it came to getting a grant for the research work he met with frustration and disappointment. He has explained: 'We tried hard to get some assistance from the Department of Health but they were not in the least interested. They were committed to POSSUM and were not prepared to provide disabled people with a choice. Yet a choice is needed because some disabled people cannot use POSSUM. We tried the charities for help, but some thought I was a crank and the only one prepared to help us was one called Invalids-at-Home, which was set up to enable permanent invalids to remain at home in greater comfort, security and independence. The chairman of this charitable trust is John Astor, Conservative M.P. for Newbury, Berkshire, and the vice-chairman, Miss Enid Hopper. The snag is that under the terms of the Trust they cannot provide for people in institutions and hospitals.'

PILOT has been available since around 1968, but at the beginning of 1972 there were only about fifty in use. A number of foreign countries, however, were taking a growing interest in the system, including the U.S.A., Canada, Sweden, Switzerland and Japan. Each system, without a typewriter, cost about £300 at the beginning of 1972.

Mr Collins has had many letters from disabled people praising his helpful machine. One woman has described it as a 'time-spending machine'. Ann Armstrong, whose problem started the whole operation, has become a first-class typist by using PILOT.

John Killick of London, completely bedridden by multiple sclerosis, is still able to lead an interesting life through the use of the digitally controlled PILOT typewriter. He has written: 'After a year spent in the irksome wilderness of hospitals it was a tremendous joy to me to be at home at last, though I had to adjust to the bitter fact that I would never again have the control or facility to stretch over a drawing board and continue in my professional life as an architect. Long days stretched ahead, but at last came the news that Invalids-at-Home were ready to lend me a fabulous electronic typewriter to add a new dimension to my life. As I had some previous experience in editing an architectural magazine, the transition from one form of creative work to another was not too difficult. I have since been able to review books on my professional subject and produce articles for specialist journals and assist in an audio-visual educational project.'

The inventor is justifiably proud of his equipment. But Collins speaks with some bitterness of the difficulties involved in trying to produce such an aid. He says: 'There's a lot of frustration – and not only because you can't do all you would like to do for disabled people. There's a lack of interest in high places. There are too many people who will take no chances, who play safe and will not spend money so that they can never be criticized by others in their organizations for spending unwisely. Meanwhile disabled people, through lack of suitable equipment, have been reduced to using pathetically inadequate means to attract attention when they require help, such as the woman pulling a piece of string to get assistance from someone upstairs . . . '

~~~~~~

Chapter Eight

The Outsiders

SID HOLLINWORTH and two friends went for a drink in Wakefield after attending a meeting for paraplegics at a local hospital. They parked their invalid cars and went to a nearby hotel in their invalid chairs. They sat at a table some yards from the bar and about ten yards from the dance floor. They thought they were out of everybody's way. But a young man was told by the landlady: 'Go and tell those men in the wheelchairs to sit against the door.' The young man did so, but said he thought it was unfair, and they decided to stay where they were. People sitting nearby agreed with them. At closing time the landlord went over to them and told them in no uncertain terms that they could not go into that room again. He added that he didn't allow dogs in because they got in the way and the same applied to people in wheelchairs.

* * *

Bill Anderson of Edinburgh had suffered from polio for fifteen years when he took up golf. He told the bulletin of the British Polio Fellowship: 'At first I had to lay down my sticks and kept losing my balance each time I swung the club.' But he persevered and by regular practice he had brought his handicap down to twenty by the end of 1971. He says about his golf: 'It has done me a power of good, kept me in excellent health and given me a good outside interest.'

* * *

A lot of disabled people admit that their handicaps make

them more depressed and moody than other men and women. Time passes with agonizing slowness, especially if they are unable to do a job of work. Well organized and absorbing leisure activities are, therefore, even more important for disabled people than for the able-bodied. An increasing amount of time, thought and money is devoted to leisure pursuits for normal families, and it is only natural that those with disabilities want to benefit from the general trend. But for the handicapped there are a host of problems to be overcome – problems ranging from means of transport to difficulties of access to places of entertainment. As a result many thousands of disabled people leave their homes for some kind of outing only a few times a year. Some have not been out of doors for years. A large number have not had a holiday for years. Trips to cinemas, theatres, sports meetings, pubs and libraries are very infrequent.

The most simple form of relaxation, and often the most pleasurable, for many people is just mixing with friends and relations. Disabled people living on their own are the most likely to have little regular contact of that sort – yet they are the very people who need it most. Much depends on the extent to which neighbours are prepared to be sociable, friendly and helpful. But the only opportunity some disabled people have of any social contact outside their own home is through clubs run by voluntary organizations – clubs where they tend to meet only other people suffering from similar disabilities.

For handicapped young people the problem of social contact with those of their own age is particularly acute. As they enter their late teens or early twenties they find themselves increasingly isolated from their able-bodied friends who go off to dances and soccer matches and begin to have affairs with the opposite sex. This is a particularly important period in which partnerships are formed that can lead to marriage – and disabled youngsters have just the same sexual desires and emotional needs as normal young people. Yet, although they usually assume that they will marry in the long term, they suffer much more frustration and worry about sexual relationships than those who are not impaired by physical or mental disabilities.

In 1964 studies were published of two groups of spastic adolescents and young adults, one living in London and the other in Scotland. The findings obviously also apply to youngsters suffering from other disabilities. In Scotland twenty-five per cent were leading a restricted social life, twenty per cent had a social life confined to their immediate family circle, and four per cent never left the house for social activities. In London it was found that most of the group made no attempt towards any social life other than that which was provided for them during their schooldays. All their energy and enterprise had been concentrated on trying to do some sort of work and many were unwilling to leave home even for a short holiday. There is clearly a need for much more guidance to be given to young disabled people about how to spend their spare time. All too often schools and local authorities concentrate all their advice and guidance on the problem of employment.

In Scotland, 186 of the 200 in the survey were of marriageable age – between sixteen and twenty-five-years – but only one male and three females were married. If they had not been disabled about eighteen per cent of the young men and thirty-three per cent of the young women would be expected to have married according to figures produced by the Registrar General. In the London survey, out of fifty-four young people aged sixteen to twenty-one as many as thirty-five appeared to have had no experience with the opposite sex at all.

As for hobbies and spare time activities, these were mostly similar to those of other young people but tended to be of the type that could be pursued alone – playing records, tape-recordings, watching television and listening to the radio.

Getting out and about to meet people is made easier if some sort of private transport is available. But car ownership among the disabled is well below the national average, and if they have a Government three-wheeled invalid car they are banned from carrying a passenger. This lack of mobility means that a telephone becomes tremendously important as a means of social contact, as well as a life-line in emergencies. The telephone, however, has been beyond the means of a great many disabled people, especially those living alone.

Mrs H. has suffered from a chronic anxiety state for the last ten years. It has prevented her from leaving her home, except for occasional walks in the night. On two occasions she has become so depressed that hospital admission has been necessary. She has no friends because of her present personality and her local doctor is not interested in her case. She cannot afford a telephone and is becoming increasingly cut off.

*   *   *

Many disabled people are deterred from seeking social contacts or entertainment away from home because of problems with incontinence and public lavatories.

A mother living in Kent has described the difficulties of her teenage daughter who suffers from spina bifida. The girl was completely incontinent until she was six and still has to reach a lavatory very quickly. On one outing with her school her wheelchair would not go through the door of a public lavatory. She had to crawl into the dirty, germ-ridden place on her hands and knees.

A sufferer from muscular dystrophy in Northants has explained how her incontinence problems are always on her mind: 'One finds oneself restricted in so many ways. So often I won't go on journeys on public transport because I think I might make a fool of myself.'

A woman in her sixties, who, like so many other elderly people, suffers from incontinence, has said: 'I find that we tend to stay at home rather than have the worry of wondering whether we shall manage if we go to a meeting or anything. It is a problem one cannot talk about to people who do not suffer in this way.'

The Government officially recognized the problem in 1968 in a circular to local authorities which said: 'Disabled people may be prevented from taking part in the active life of the community simply by the absence of suitable toilet facilities. For example, they may be deterred from spending a day at the seaside or an afternoon shopping if they cannot be sure of finding a public convenience which they can use. Severely handicapped people confined to wheelchairs need a W.C. compartment large enough to take both their wheelchair and someone to help them.' Some local authorities took note and action. Many appear to have disregarded the circular.

Incontinence can afflict people who are not disabled in any other way. A woman in her mid forties, attractive but desperately lonely, has explained how this problem has ruined her life: 'I feel lonely and unwanted and because I am such a fastidious person I feel bitter that this thing has happened to me. I even took an overdose of tablets last year because I couldn't face it.'

But many people who have been in the depths of despair have been helped to lead a more normal life again by advice about special clothing and equipment from bodies like the Disabled Living Foundation.

Holidays are virtually unknown to hundreds of thousands of disabled people. Sally Sainsbury, in the course of a survey (*Registered As Disabled*, 1970) of problems confronting disabled people, discovered that thirty-nine per cent of the people in her sample had not had a holiday for six years or more.

Voluntary organizations and local authorities provide some holidays for disabled people.

By 1971, holidays for 1,100 disabled people were being provided each year by the Winged Fellowship Trust – thanks to the drive and dedication of a remarkable woman, Mrs Joan Brander. Her work in this field began in 1958. In that year, as a member of the Women's Royal Voluntary Service, she assisted in taking a group of disabled people from Bermondsey, London, to a holiday camp at Grange Farm, Essex. She had come to realize that many very severely disabled people never got a holiday – nor did the members of their families who looked after them.

Within a year or two the W.R.V.S. were faced with growing waiting lists for their Grange Farm holidays – despite the fact that the camp was not well equipped to cater for disabled people. Joan Brander wanted to improve the camp and if possible build a large, well equipped holiday home. But she could get no help from the Department of Health or local authorities. Finally she was given £1,200 by the *People* – the Sunday newspaper that has campaigned strongly over the years on behalf of disabled people. The donation enabled her to build a special lavatory block and a bathroom at Grange

Farm. But the camp came nowhere near to meeting the real need.

Joan Brander took her next decisive action to meet that need as the result of a particularly sad case. A young woman had agreed on marrying her husband that they would provide a home for her sister and sister-in-law, who were both suffering from progressively disabling diseases. She and her husband knew that they could never expect a holiday by themselves and that caring for these two handicapped women would leave them little time for leisure. But they could not have been expected to see just how extraordinarily difficult life would become for them. At first they were assisted by one of their mothers who did the housework and other chores, but she became bedridden with arthritis. Next, the husband contracted a rare disease of the hands which left him so helpless that his wife had to do everything for him. Then her only brother became paralysed as the result of a car crash. By middle age she had become wage earner and nurse to five disabled people. She got some assistance from the local authority – home helps, for example. But what she desperately needed was a holiday. And it was the fact that she could not assist this hard-pressed woman that prompted Joan Brander to launch a more ambitious holiday scheme.

She recalls: 'I was choked by this situation. I had been to the Health Ministry and to the local authorities but no one would give me any money. And they call it the Welfare State!' She decided to start a charity to raise funds and with the help of a few friends and her husband she formed the Winged Fellowship Trust. It got its name from the remark of one disabled person who, on being given a holiday, said: 'It's like being given wings.' The Trust raised enough money to buy and equip Crabhill House, Surrey.

Although she started her holiday schemes at a camp, Joan Brander does not believe that these are the best places to send severely disabled and incontinent men and women as they are not usually equipped or designed to cater for their special problems. She cites the case of a disabled man, weighing twenty stone, paralysed from the armpits down, and doubly incontinent. He had been in a good job and was able to buy a large second hand car in which to drive himself about. His local authority also added to his independence by providing him with some good aids and equipment. As a result his wife, a frail woman, never has to lift him. But when the local authority sent the couple on a holiday to a camp at Skegness they found it was no pleasure at all. There were no hoists and equipment and no lavatories attached to the chalets. The husband decided that it was unfair to his wife so they stayed only one night. And they have not had a holiday since.

Another problem about such camps is that relatives must accompany the disabled person, although it is often these other members of the family who badly need a period on their own if they are to avoid a breakdown. This problem is illustrated by another of Joan Brander's cases. One day in 1970 she received a phone call from a woman who sobbed that the doctor had ordered her disabled husband to be sent to hospital on the ground that she was unable to look after him at home. Tired and physically weak she had dropped her husband on three occasions when trying to help him to the lavatory. On the last occasion he had injured his head. If that woman had been given the opportunity to take a holiday on her own she might have built up enough strength to carry on looking after her husband at home – so saving the taxpayers the considerable cost of keeping him in hospital.

The work of the Winged Fellowship Trust has attracted attention abroad and brought inquiries from Scandinavian and East European countries among others. But in Sweden, Denmark and Holland the governments are doing much more than the British Government to help with this important problem. The Swedish Government, for example, has spent over £1 million on a showpiece hotel for disabled people. The intention is to encourage others to follow suit. Mrs Brander regrets that Britain has no such showplace.

She says: 'I wrote to a number of very wealthy people asking for help. They have replied to the effect: "That's old hat. People are always doing something for the disabled. Let's do something new."'

Apart from the work of the voluntary organizations and charities there are schemes organized by local authorities. The

Department of Health and Social Security had a survey into such schemes carried out by its Social Science Research Unit. Some two hundred authorities were approached of which thirty-six had no scheme and ten failed to reply. In the 158 authorities which provided information on schemes a total of 56,000 people received special holidays in 1969. The cost was an average of £13 each, of which the disabled contributed on average £3 each and the authorities £10. The most serious problem was finding suitable accommodation. The next was transport.

One difficulty in planning vacations in holiday camps or hotels used by normal families is the belief that some other holidaymakers do not like to see a lot of disabled people about. A hotel director from Cornwall told a conference on holidays organized by the Central Council for the Disabled in December 1970, that this had not been his experience in Bude. He admitted, however, that when he and his family had received their first coach-load of disabled people they had watched with dismay as crutches, wheelchairs and other contraptions were unloaded from the boot and the guests were wheeled or carried or hobbled into the hotel. In no time at all, however, everyone had settled down happily. He also found that the physically handicapped and old age pensioners were far easier to please and much more appreciative of anything done for them than the ordinary individual. He said: 'These people had an acute sense of values and their main trouble was, perhaps, that often they did not expect, and certainly did not demand, many of those things to which they were entitled.'

More and more disabled men, women and children are taking part in sport and physical recreation – much to the amazement of many able-bodied people. They swim, play golf, ride horses, play basket-ball, take part in archery contests and many other sports. At archery, bowls, table tennis and some other recreations they often excel over those who suffer from no disabilities. They derive tremendous benefits – both physical and psychological – from such activities. The Disabled Living Foundation, which carried out an inquiry into physical recreation, cited the following cases:

A man severely disabled through a malformed spine had been hidden by his parents for thirty-five years. He had never worked and never been for a holiday. Later he was given a mechanized wheelchair and fishing rods. This man now has a job and spends fishing holidays at the seaside. His life has been revolutionized.

A young man fitted with artificial legs resumed his previous hobby – mountain climbing. He tackled Tryfan in Snowdonia accompanied by one able-bodied friend. The climb took him five hours. Part of the time he was struggling through deep snow and he completed the last stretch on all fours.

Special equipment has been devised to enable disabled people to take part in sports – such as reinforced boots for skaters with weak legs and waterproof coverings for swimmers with artificial legs.

The world's finest purpose-built sports stadium for disabled athletes is at the Spinal Injuries Centre at Stoke Mandeville, Buckinghamshire. Director of this remarkable centre is Sir Ludwig Guttman, who introduced a new type of treatment based on sport for paraplegics and other handicapped people. He has shown that sport has a great therapeutic value and can restore strength and co-ordination to a disabled person. Apart from training the body it also gives patients a new interest, helps to prevent boredom and can play an important part in restoring self confidence.

The first Stoke Mandeville Games for the Paralysed were held in 1948. There were sixteen competitors. Over the years this sports festival has steadily grown and has attracted competitors from all over the world. Up to 1971 over fifty countries had been represented. Ethiopia has been represented at a recent games by Abebe Bikila, a former captain in the bodyguard of Emperor Haile Selassie. He suffered a spinal injury in a car crash in 1969 and became a patient at Stoke Mandeville. He took part in the archery contest in the games but he is better known as a long distance runner: he holds two Olympic Gold Medals for the marathon.

The Stoke Mandeville Games won an award themselves in 1956. The Olympic Committee awarded this extraordinary sports meeting the Fearnley Cup for outstanding achievement in the Olympic ideal. In that year Guttman explained his purpose to the competitors in these words: 'The aim of the Stoke Mandeville Games is to unite paralysed men and women from all parts of the world in an international sports movement and your spirit of true sportsmanship today will give hope and inspiration to thousands of paralysed people. No greater contribution can be made to society by the paralysed than to help, through the medium of sport, to further friendship and understanding amongst nations.'

Events at the games include basketball, fencing, swimming, table tennis, weight lifting, javelin, archery, shot putting and wheelchair racing. High standards are achieved. In archery the women have produced a paraplegic record of 2,239 compared to a world record of 2,332. Up to 1971, the international paraplegic record for the shot was 10·44 metres and the fastest freestyle swim over 50 metres was 36·5 seconds.

Most of the governing bodies for sport have done something to help disabled sportsmen and women and some local authorities have a good record in providing money, premises, transport, equipment and classes.

Disabled people usually prefer to mix with able-bodied people at clubs and sports centres. But unless the premises are purpose-built they usually encounter difficulties with steps, narrow doors and lavatories and awkward corridors. The Disabled Living Foundation's inquiry concluded that disabled people were not being provided with adequate opportunities for physical recreation. It recommended that so far as facilities were concerned it would be simpler and cheaper to cater for the needs of handicapped people in existing premises and those in course of construction rather than make separate provision later. It favoured disabled and non-disabled people using the same premises and participating together. This view is supported by a lot of disabled people themselves. They point out that if they meet only other handicapped people at clubs they all tend to talk about their impairments and operations. Mixing with able-bodied people helps to take their minds off their problems and opens up new interests.

Music plays an important part in the lives of many disabled men and women. A large number of handicapped people are keen to play an instrument and if this enthusiasm wanes in later life they enjoy listening to records and concerts.

Joanne Seymour, in her early teens, has been disabled by polio since she was one year old. She is a keen musician and is learning to play the clarinet. She has also competed at archery, table tennis and other events at the Stoke Mandeville Games. She is a patrol leader in the Girl Guides and has been awarded the Girl Guide Star of Merit for courage in illness.

Mrs Joan Skipper, another polio victim, took up music at the age of twelve to compensate for not being able to take part in active sports. Now she is one of the best known singing and drama teachers in Coventry.

The Disabled Living Foundation, in a report on music for the handicapped, told of a disabled woman in her mid forties who travelled a five-mile return journey by taxi to attend her weekly piano lesson.

Singing is another important leisure activity for the disabled. They have formed a number of choirs and some of these are assisted by local authorities.

Miss Monica Young told a conference on music organized by the Disabled Living Foundation in 1970 about the important part music had played in her life. She contracted polio at twelve and on leaving hospital found she could no longer play the piano. Her family encouraged her to take up singing instead. After early lessons from friends she went to a London teacher. This meant travelling to London by train – sitting in the guard's van in her wheelchair. The railway guards were a great help in heaving her wheelchair up and down steps and in and out of the van. They took a great interest in her singing. But she told the conference that in trying to join choirs and generally take part in musical activities disabled people met the ever-present problem of access.

'Sometimes when one tries to join a choir or enter a competitive festival there are architectural barriers. The imposing flight of steps, so beloved by architects of former times, can mean exclusion to someone confined to a wheelchair.'

Some concert halls might just as well carry a notice saying: 'Disabled people keep out.' The same applies to most theatres and cinemas, bingo halls, libraries and art galleries. A man who had planned a Christmas cinema treat for a party of disabled children was told by the manager that he could not permit wheelchairs in his large West End cinema. Another West End manager explained to a disabled person that he would like to let him enter in a wheelchair but this was forbidden by local authority fire regulations.

The problem of access was highlighted in ironic fashion in 1971 when a film entitled 'The Raging Moon' on the subject of the disabled was shown at the ABC 2 cinema in London's Shaftesbury Avenue. Neither the author Peter Marshall, nor one of the stars, Michael Flanders, was able to attend the film showing. The reason: they both use wheelchairs and the cinema was inaccessible to this basic piece of equipment for disabled people.

Chapter Nine

~~~~~~

Race Against Time

AT 11.05 a.m. on Friday, 5 December, 1969, Alfred Morris rose in the House of Commons to move the Second Reading of the Chronically Sick and Disabled Persons Bill. He began by declaring that it dealt with many problems, all of them intensely human, but it had a single intention: to extend the welfare, improve the status, and enhance the dignity of chronically sick and disabled people. It had been put to the sponsors that ideas, even good ideas, for helping the disabled ceased to be good if they cost money. The counter argument was simply that there might even be a net saving in public money if increasing home care and welfare services eased the strain on the hospital service and if increased mobility and employment opportunities made the disabled less dependent on State aid.

The philosophy behind the Bill was put to the Commons in these words: 'What most disabled people want more than anything else is to lessen their dependence on other people, to get on with living their own lives as normally as they can in their own homes among their own family and, wherever possible, to have the opportunity of contributing to industry and society as fully as their abilities allow.

'Investment in people, disabled people no less than fit and strong and fortunate people, is much the best of all investments.'

How had Morris and his helpers sought to implement that philosophy in the light of the problems they had uncovered and the political realities of getting a Bill through Parliament? The Act which reached the Statute Book six months later on 29 May 1970, differed very little in substance from the Bill originally introduced. The passage of this extraordinary measure through Parliament, however, was not without its moments of tension and drama, its disappointments and back-stairs deals.

The key to the whole new deal is to be found in the very first section. Under this authorities are given the duty of finding out how many chronically sick and disabled people are living in their areas. Most organizations working to help the disabled had agreed that there should be such a register, subject only to a person's willingness to have his name included. Indeed, such a register already existed for blind people. Under the National Assistance Act 1948 local authorities were obliged to keep a register of handicapped people who applied for aid. But this provided a big loophole for those councils who were not anxious to help disabled people. If they failed to advertise their services they could restrict the numbers applying for aid. It was up to the local authorities themselves to decide how good a job they would do. The result was a wide gap between the registers kept and services offered by good authorities and those provided by the less conscientious. The Morris Bill aimed to change all that. It aimed, moreover, to add a new dimension to the welfare state. No longer was it to be good enough for authorities to provide aid for the needy who came knocking at the town hall door. A new obligation was being put on local councils: the obligation to go out and find all the chronically sick and disabled who could benefit from the support of the welfare services. This was an entirely new concept and a dramatic change in the law. Its importance has tended to overshadow other important provisions in a very wide-ranging Bill.

The next provision of the Bill was closely linked to the first. Local authorities were to be obliged to discover the needs of people registered as disabled and provide a wide range of services for them. These ranged from practical help in the home to radio, T.V. and library facilities; a telephone;

recreational facilities; help in taking holidays; meals at home or elsewhere; transport for recreation, treatment or jobs; and adaptations to the home. Before the Act, authorities could choose whether to provide certain services. The Act makes it a legal duty.

In an attempt to tackle the housing needs of the disabled, the Act places an entirely new duty on local authorities to take such needs fully into account when planning future housing developments. In submitting new housing proposals to the Government, they now have to show that they have had regard to the special needs of the long-term sick and disabled.

The problem of access to buildings, from municipal offices to cinemas, is dealt with in another section. This places a duty on the owner of any new building to which the public are to be admitted, whether on payment or otherwise, to provide both means of access and proper facilities for the disabled. Access for the disabled has to be into the building, within the building, in the car parks and into the lavatories. It was made clear in the Parliamentary debates on the Bill that the *caveat* about 'practicable and reasonable' that was entered was only to exclude very small existing buildings like corner shops. The intention of Parliament was that ultimately every public and social building would have to be accessible to and usable by disabled people before planning permission was given.

Several other sections deal with various aspects of access. Local authorities must provide, as far as practicable, for the needs of disabled people in public sanitary conveniences – and these must be adequately signposted. Owners of hotels, restaurants, cinemas, theatres and other social buildings, who are required to provide sanitary facilities, will also have to make provision for the disabled.

Access to schools and universities is tackled by a section which constitutes an important amendment to the Education Act 1944. It is of benefit alike to disabled children, students and teachers. It states that facilities for access to such places of learning, including teacher-training colleges, must be provided for the disabled. Parking and sanitary conveniences must be provided, too.

Action to ensure that disabled people get a seat at the top table when issues affecting them are being discussed at Government level is taken by several sections dealing with the councils and committees that advise Ministers and state-owned industries on the making of social policy. The Act provides for disabled people, and those closely connected with them, to sit on a range of committees set up to advise ministers and public bodies on such subjects as housing, pensions, employment and industrial injuries.

The deep concern about young chronically sick and disabled people being housed in hospital wards for geriatrics is dealt with in another important section. Hospital boards must now ensure that such young people are not cared for in wards normally reserved for elderly men and women, often senile and near to death. The boards must now inform the Secretary of State of every case of a young person detained in such a ward. The minister, in turn, must report to Parliament each year. The purpose: to bring this grave problem to an early end. Local authorities must also provide similar information on young and homeless disabled people held in residential homes for those over sixty-five.

The Act goes on to provide a number of measures aimed at improving the mobility of the chronically sick and disabled. There is a provision to extend local authority chiropody services to those under sixty-five. Restrictions on the use of invalid carriages on footways, including electrically-powered wheelchairs, are lifted. This part of the Act can be of great help to thalidomide children and other very severely disabled youngsters. And a new national scheme to help disabled drivers and disabled passengers with parking problems is introduced. Under this scheme, all local authorities must issue a badge for display on vehicles used by disabled people living in their areas and such badges will be recognized by all other authorities.

The fight to get improved equipment for disabled people is given new impetus by what is one of the most far-reaching provisions of the Act. This obliges the Secretary of State to report to Parliament each year on the research and development work undertaken on equipment that may be of use to the disabled, particularly with regard to improving their mobility. This improves Parliament's scrutiny of the Government and means that there will be an annual debate in the Commons on action being taken to help the disabled get around.

Important changes in the law dealing with war pensions appeals are also made. The result will be to make the process of appeals up to six times quicker than before.

Help for the deaf is provided by obliging the Secretary of State to present evidence to the Medical Research Council on the need to set up an Institute of Hearing Research.

The special education required by children suffering from certain severely disabling handicaps is dealt with by further amendments to the Education Act 1944. These aim to help deaf-blind, dyslexic and autistic children as well as those suffering from other forms of early childhood psychosis. Local education authorities must now report to the Secretary of State on the educational services they are providing for such children, and the Act states that wherever possible such facilities must be provided by the local authority in its own schools. These provisions of the Act are deeply important for the future of many of the most severely disabled children in Britain.

Twenty-two of the twenty-nine sections of the Act came into force on 29 August 1970. Other sections came into operation later. But Section (1), enforcing the identification of the disabled living at home, did not come into operation until 1 October 1971. This long delay caused much trouble and disappointment, for Section (1) was the Bill's master key to the main problem of the missing million.

The original Bill that came up for Second Reading in December had several proposals that were dropped in face of Government opposition. They included a thoroughgoing review of the vehicle service for disabled people and, in particular, the provision in all appropriate cases of a four-wheeled vehicle to replace the much criticised three-wheeled invalid tricycle. Another clause dealt with the self-defeating earnings rule for the wives of men who were long-term sick. This clause was later taken up by the Tory Government and has now become law.

Within a few minutes of the opening of the debate John Temple, Tory M.P. for Chester, rose to point to a serious gap in the Bill. There was no new definition of chronically sick and disabled persons. This was a problem of complexity on which David Weitzman, M.P., was already at work. At that stage the nearest the drafting had got to solving the problem was an attempt to define the younger chronic sick in what was then Clause 20. But no one spoke against the measure. In fact, those who took part in the day-long debate were mostly drawn from the small all-party band of back-benchers who had campaigned over the years for a better deal for disabled people.

Neil Marten spoke of the need for a four-wheeled vehicle, especially for haemophiliacs; Jack Ashley spoke in particular of the problems of the deaf; John Astor referred to the economic problems facing the disabled, of their fight against the twin forces of increased living costs and reduced earning capacity; Lewis Carter-Jones on the need to harness technology.

Laurie Pavitt made a moving personal reference to the problem of deafness from which he had suffered for years. Explaining that the needs of the deaf were not fully understood by society he commented:

'Members of the public do not appreciate the sense of isolation which deafness can bring. One of the saddest places in the world for a person with hearing loss is the Tea Room of the House of Commons. One is not lonely when by oneself but one is lonely when surrounded by friends and colleagues with mutual interests and yet outside. It is not possible to join in the gossip and laughter. One worries if there is any criticism of the apparent stand-offishness because one dare not participate in what is going on.'

The official Tory Party attitude was put by Paul Dean, from the Opposition Front Bench. In view of the fact that a General Election could not be far ahead, his words were of special interest. Dean welcomed the Bill 'in principle' and hoped it would go on to Committee where it could be con-

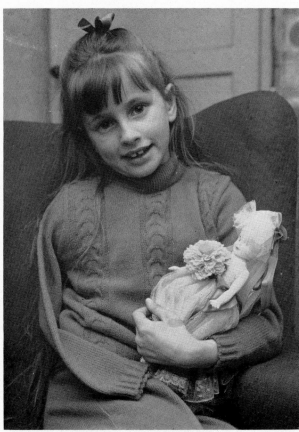

Debbie Leigh, of Oldham, cuddles her doll in her left arm. Her right arm was removed by surgeons nine months before this picture was taken. Debbie is a victim of cancer. One day her mother took her on her knee and told her: 'Darling, unless they take your arm off you are going to die.'

Volunteers helping to bath a severely handicapped man on holiday at a Winged Fellowship Trust holiday centre.

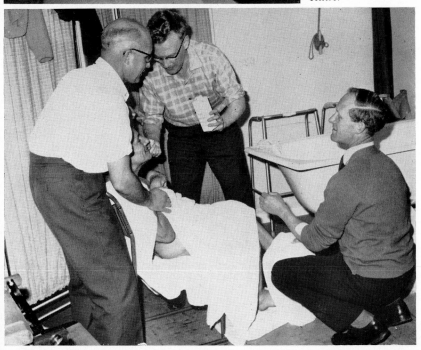

A child tends her miniature garden, an absorbing pastime for a disabled youngster, and one of many activities encouraged by the Disabled Living Foundation.

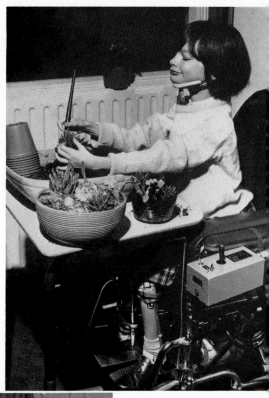

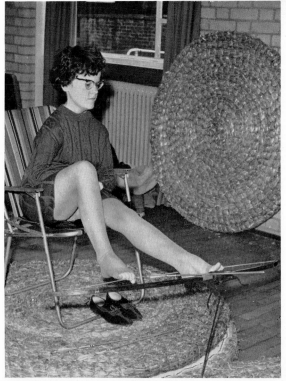

A disabled woman with a go pair of feet has her own meth with the bow and arrow. Han capped men and women ha good results at archery, one of most popular sports for disabled.

sidered in detail. He also hoped that there would not be too many amendments at Committee Stage and that the Bill would speedily reach the Statute Book.

He was particularly pleased that there was a clause dealing with the earnings rule for the wife of a sick man – a clause which, as we have seen, was not to survive the Committee Stage. Dean pointed out that a wife who went out to work to try to keep the home together was allowed to earn only £3 2s. a week before losing all her allowance. 'Surely we want to encourage such a wife to support her family and be able to look after the home.'

The Government's attitude was expressed publicly for the first time by Dr John Dunwoody, Under Secretary of State at Richard Crossman's huge Department of Health and Social Security. It may have been an oversight that he did not go as far as Paul Dean in expressing the hope that the Bill would reach the Statute Book, but he welcomed the measure and hoped the Commons would give it a Second Reading. There was, in fact, throughout his speech a note of caution – a note that must have echoed some of the coolness and reservations of the absent Secretary of State. He said that clauses dealing with social security benefits – such as the earnings rule for wives of sick men – would have to be considered in the light of the National Superannuation Bill, which his department was to introduce into the Commons shortly. Moreover, as work was now well ahead with the Government's Social Survey on the disabled and handi-capped, they should show patience until the whole exercise was more clearly comprehensible. It would not be in the interests of the services or their beneficiaries to rush into premature conclusions ... A decisive consideration, too, was the problem of resources. Strict limits on the growth of public spending had been imposed as part of the policy to get the economy right. Financial resources could not be stretched indefinitely. The absence of definitions also raised difficulties.

'Who are the chronically sick and disabled?' asked Dunwoody, 'Like the elephant, they are easy to recognize but hard to describe.'

Dunwoody warned that some of the matters would have to

be further examined 'to achieve a practical result' but he nevertheless hoped the Commons would give the Bill a Second Reading. The Commons did just that.

The first Commons hurdle had been cleared but there was now an enormous amount of work to do in tidying up the hastily put-together measure before it entered the Committee Stage, where M.P.s would consider it in detail, line by line. Luckily there was no problem in forming a committee of M.P.s who were dedicated to getting something done. It included such members of the Commons pressure group as Ashley, Astor, Carter-Jones, Maurice Macmillan, Fred Evans, Neil Marten, Laurie Pavitt, Jim Prior, John Golding, Dame Irene Ward, David Weitzmann and Sir Clive Bossom. The Christmas recess was only a few weeks ahead and this was to provide a much-needed breathing space for knocking the Bill into shape. There would be time for only one meeting of the Committee before then. That was fortunate in view of the large amount of drafting to be done. Morris had to limp along as best as he could to the Christmas break. Behind the scenes he was involved in continual negotiation and wrangling with members of the numerous Government departments affected. The Housing Department now became very constructive in helping to polish up the clauses on housing and access. This no doubt had something to do with the late Arthur Skeffington's growing interest in the Bill. There was also the fact that Reginald Freeson, another of the Parliamentary Secretaries at the Ministry, who had joined the Committee on the Bill, was a man of considerable determination and dedication when it came to improving the lot of people in special need. The Education Department, however, at first tended to drag its feet.

The Committee Stage tussle began on Wednesday, 17 December. Because work was still going on to improve the drafting of the early clauses in the Bill, Morris, with the support of the chairman, Sir Myer Galpern, asked the Committee to take the apparently eccentric course of virtually beginning at the end. The Committee's discussions started on one of the last clauses in the Bill – the one put forward by the then Ministry of Transport to allow certain types of invalid carriages to be used on the footpath. No better clause could have been chosen in terms of starting the Committee's work in an atmosphere of broad agreement. But as soon as the Committee moved to the next clause it ran into trouble with the Government and had its first public sign that there were disputes behind the scenes in Whitehall.

Technology Minister Anthony Wedgwood Benn had helped to draw up the clause which proposed that his department should produce an annual report on the progress made in applying science and technology to assist the disabled. This was a clause that began life as a scribbled note on the back of an envelope following a conversation between Morris and Benn in the Tea Room of the House of Commons.

A report by the British Medical Association Planning unit had recently castigated the artificial limb and appliance industry. It had been accused of presenting an improbable combination of the disadvantages of monopoly, centralized supply and technical backwardness. The industry was also accused of failing to exploit recent developments in the field. It was alleged that this had caused Britain to fall behind other developed countries in the use of the plastic and prefabricated prosthesis that permits individual fitting, immediate supply and the economies of mass production. There was clearly an urgent need to review the situation. But when John Dunwoody rose to speak it soon became obvious that the Health Department did not like the idea of such a report. Clearly the power struggle between Whitehall departments that had been the death of many good ideas in the past was going to be particularly troublesome on legislation involving no less than eleven ministries.

Dunwoody asserted that the research and development work being done was largely related to his department rather than to any others. He added that his department already published two reports a year, but he promised that they would in future contain more detail on technical progress.

The Committee was due to hold its next meeting immediately after the Christmas recess. Meanwhile, Morris, living a hand-to-mouth existence in improving clauses of the

Bill while dealing with an enormous correspondence from disabled people, was beginning to fear that the whole operation would prove to be too much for him. He had visions of the whole project crashing about his ears because of the growing administrative difficulties. Apart from the continual struggle with Whitehall, he was inundated with letters from all over Britain from people anxious to help or to unburden their personal problems. At one stage he received 1,100 letters in two days, many of them from severely disabled people with appalling difficulties. Then, just before the Christmas break, he was invited to a Commons lunch in honour of seven former Ministers of Health. Seated next to him was Duncan Guthrie, Director of the Central Council for the Disabled, whom he was meeting for the first time. He told Guthrie of his difficulties. Guthrie readily offered help, especially with much-needed secretarial work to cope with the mounting flood of correspondence. A new and vital source of aid had arrived – just in time. From then on, Morris never again had cause to fear that the Bill would fail because of his own administrative problems.

Members of other organizations for disabled people were doing their bit by keeping up the pressure on Ministers and M.P.s. About thirty disabled drivers drove through the snow of that December from Hyde Park to the Commons in their invalid tricycles. A deputation from the little procession went in to see Dunwoody to urge the Government to support the Bill and, in particular, to provide the disabled with small cars instead of tricycles. Dunwoody himself, when a back-bencher, had once said that it was wrong to expect disabled people to drive around in these 'abysmal vehicles'. He was less outspoken now and the deputation left without any promise of action to replace the tricycles.

With the aid of ministers, however, not least of Dunwoody, the Bill continued to take shape in Committee after Christmas and on 4 February the Government took an important step without which the Bill would have failed in its purpose. Through a Money Resolution in Parliament it gave authority for money to be spent to implement the measure. That was not the same as saying that a definite sum of money would

be spent. But it was an important – indeed indispensable –
step in that direction. It meant that a Rate Support Grant
could be paid by the Central Government in support of the
new local services for which the Bill provided. As was later
shown by the reaction of the local officials who spoke in
ignorance of the financial provision, much of the Act would
rapidly have become a dead duck without the money
resolution.

The Bill completed its Committee Stage and on 20 March
came up for Third Reading in the Commons. Morris,
speaking with the gift of foresight, warned that 'time may
prove to be our keenest adversary in our efforts to complete
the remaining stages . . . ' Laurie Pavitt, with some exas-
peration, declared that it was high time the Government
appointed a minister with sole responsibility for the chronically sick and disabled. They now had twelve senior ministers
concerned with the problem tackled by the Bill!

The Bill had, in fact, completed its Commons stages in
what would normally have been good time and was ready to
be debated by the Lords immediately after Easter. But
speculation now began about the possibility of an early
General Election. If Harold Wilson decided to try Labour's
luck at the polls in June, it would be touch and go whether
the Bill would complete the course in time.

Lord Longford, a recent ex-member of the Wilson Cabinet,
had agreed to sponsor the Bill in the Lords. He had resigned
from the Cabinet over economies in the education service
and, as a former Leader of the House, was both highly
qualified in procedure and much respected in the House of
Lords.

When the Bill came up for Second Reading in the Lords
on 9 April the occasion was marked by a very unusual re-
arrangement of furniture in the ornate red and gold chamber.
The first row of the crossbenches was removed to make way
for what became known as the 'wheelchair brigade' or the
'mobile bench'. This was composed of four disabled members
of the House who were determined to attend in their wheelchairs to take part in the debates on the measure. One of
these was Baroness Masham, whose barony in the New

Year's Honours List had made her, at thirty-four the youngest Life Peeress. She had decided to make her maiden speech on the Bill; she could speak from experience as she had been paralysed from the waist down since a hunting accident twelve years before. The others were Lady Darcy de Knayth, a young peeress and mother, who had been paralysed since a car crash in 1964 in which her husband was killed; Lord Ingleby, a polio victim; and Lord Crawshaw, paralysed since a riding accident in 1954.

The Bill received a Second Reading and moved on to Committee Stage as speculation continued to grow about a June General Election. Political commentators had always assumed that Harold Wilson would call an election as soon as the public opinion polls suggested that he had a good chance of winning. Those polls were now moving in Labour's favour following Mr Roy Jenkins's Budget.

As Morris and his friends in the Commons surveyed the state of play in the Lords some of them began to get uneasy. Such was the zeal of the peers that fifteen pages of amendments had been tabled for the Committee Stage, due to begin on 30 April. Lord Oakshott, a Tory peer, appealed to their Lordships not to strive too hard for perfection in case the Bill was lost. Lord Longford, however, was not in favour of a rushed job. He argued that the House must do its duty properly. He had read in the press that the peers were in danger of destroying the Bill, but he strongly repudiated that suggestion. There were some, in fact, who still believed that the Prime Minister would not throw overboard a mass of important Government legislation – almost a full year's Parliamentary work – when there was no reason for calling a General Election apart from the enticing look of the public opinion polls.

Meanwhile the Government, in these last stages of the Bill, was showing itself reluctant to accept the attempt to get full identification of all the disabled. Baroness Serota, Minister of State for Health and Social Security, told the Committee: 'We see the greatest difficulties in regard to what would amount to a 100 per cent registration. There are clearly financial difficulties . . . Equally it would make heavy demands on the staff of the authorities concerned. Further, in some people's minds there are philosophical objections. There are those who could regard this duty placed upon the local authority as an intervention into their private lives.' Yet in the Commons, Morris had emphasized again and again that full registration would be subject both to confidentiality and the voluntary agreement of the disabled.

When the Committee met again on 15 May even Lord Longford had decided that the General Election fever was not just idle press speculation. He declared: 'Every reader of the newspapers this morning will assume that there is going to be a General Election in June – or thereabouts. I feel that we should not behave and fight on as though nothing had happened. There must be some adjustment in our attitude, although I am not suggesting that there should be unconditional surrender.'

It was clear that the Government was indeed getting ready to abandon a mass of legislation in its belief that the public was ready to vote it back for another term. Tory Party leaders were not unduly distressed by the prospect of much of this legislation being lost. But Lord Balniel, with the backing of the Shadow Cabinet and speaking as Tory Health spokesman in the Commons, caused a flurry in Labour's ranks by publicly pledging that if the Morris Bill were lost the Conservatives would bring it in as a Government measure immediately after the election. If the debates on the Bill had produced no other effect, they had at least alerted all leading politicians to the fact that the disabled and their families added up to several million people – and several million votes.

The *Sunday Times*, which under the editorship of Harold Evans had become a major crusading force on behalf of the disabled, warned on 17 May that the Bill must not be lost.

'We favour a June election because the country is in limbo, with the Government reduced to tactical manoeuvring. There would be few regrettable legislative casualties. Mrs Castle's Industrial Relations Bill is entirely dispensable; indeed the Bill most worth pushing through the final stages is not a Government Bill at all but Mr Alfred Morris's Private Member's Bill for the Disabled.'

The cliff-hanger in the Lords had by now attracted the attention of the whole of the Press. Harold Wilson too, had got the message. He made it known that whatever else might have to be abandoned the Morris Bill would be given enough priority to ensure that it reached the Statute Book. To complete their discussion of the Bill in time, the Lords even met after dinner one night – a sign of real emergency.

On 27 May the Bill returned to the Commons to enable M.P.s to debate the Lords' amendments. Winding up the debate Dr Dunwoody described the Bill as a 'compassionate and civilized Charter . . . '

On 29 May the Bill received the Royal Assent – the last measure to become law before Parliament dispersed to the hustings.

Among the Bills abandoned by the Government was the massive National Superannuation measure of Secretary of State Richard Crossman.

~~~~~~

Chapter Ten

The Feet Draggers

T H E jubilant but somewhat dazed Conservatives who swept to power under Edward Heath in the General Election of June 18 inherited, among other things, the Chronically Sick and Disabled Persons Act, 1970.

One of the surprises in Prime Minister Heath's new Cabinet list was the appointment of Sir Keith Joseph as Secretary of State for Health and Social Security. Lord Balniel, who had served as Shadow minister in this field, was made Minister of State, Defence. Sir Keith's last post in Opposition had been that of spokesman on trade and industry where he had made a reputation as an advocate of bracing right-wing policies with the emphasis on competitive efficiency. But he had always shown great interest in social policy and was expected to combine in his new office a practical, hard-headed approach with a deep sense of compassion.

The success of the Morris Bill in reaching the Statute Book on the very last day of the old Parliament had produced a momentary sense of triumph among the M.P.s and peers who had championed the cause. The achievement had been pushed out of the headlines by the opening of the General Election, but many disabled people all over the country believed that they had been presented with a charter from which benefits would soon start to flow.

The news that the Royal Assent had been given to the Bill

on 29 May had brought these comments from leading campaigners among the voluntary organizations:

Duncan Guthrie, of the Central Council for the Disabled, declared: 'It will be the first Act on the Statute Book for all disabled people and it is a basis for their rights in much the same way as Magna Carta is the basis for the rights of the British people generally.'

Mary Greaves, Director of the Disablement Income Group, said: 'As a disabled person, the importance of this Bill is the underlying philosophy: the integration of the disabled person into society. The great thing I want is to be ordinary, to be part of society, to go to places, whether to school, college, or to see friends . . . The Bill is forwarding the integration of disabled people as ordinary citizens, not as second-class citizens.'

The sense of triumph was short-lived. Two months after the Conservatives had won the General Election and twelve days before important sections of the Act was due to become operative Sir Keith Joseph issued a circular to local authorities. It dealt with what Morris and many of his supporters had regarded as a crucial matter – the need for a complete register of the disabled: the identification of the needy as a first step to providing the assistance available under the new Act.

The circular of 17 August said: 'It is not a requirement of the Section (1) that authorities should attempt 100 per cent identification and registration of the handicapped.'

Under Section (1) it had been made a duty for local authorities first to search out all the disabled in their areas; and second, to give them full information on all the services available to them. By his interpretation Sir Keith was attempting to blow a hole right through it. He went on to provide the damaging and incredible explanation that 'complete registration of the handicapped would be so great a diversion of resources of manpower and money that there would be nothing left over to meet the needs of those registered.'

Instead, the minister proposed that local authorities should assess the overall size and nature of the demand for services under the Act with a fair degree of accuracy by the use of sampling and survey techniques.

Why had the Government adopted this restrictive approach? There can be no doubt that Whitehall was appalled by the financial implications of a 100 per cent register. With the Treasury calling the tune a new dimension was not yet to be added to the so-called Welfare State. The idea that local authorities should be obliged to seek out people in need now seemed in danger of remaining an ideal. The circular soon came under fire from Labour M.P.s. Yet is there any reason to believe that a Labour Secretary of State would have acted differently? In the last stages of debate on the Bill in the House of Lords, Baroness Serota, speaking for the Wilson Government, had stressed that the administration saw the greatest difficulties in regard to a 100 per cent identification. She referred to financial, manpower and other difficulties.

More disappointments were to follow. By the autumn of 1970 complaints began to grow that some local authorities were being tardy in implementing the Act. The welfare sections, dealing with provision of practical help in the home, leisure facilities, the installation of telephones and many other aids for disabled people, had come into operation on 29 August. Sections dealing with access to public buildings were due to take effect on 29 November. Yet some local authorities were acting as though they were unaware of their new responsibilities.

At that time some of the local offices of the Department of Health and Social Security were unaware of the provisions of the Act. Two of these offices even wrote to the Central Council for the Disabled requesting details of the measure.

Letters of complaint and disappointment from disabled people and their families began to flow in to M.P.s and voluntary organizations. A typical complaint: 'I have been to my local welfare office and they said they had never heard of the Act.' Another alleged: 'The Medical Officer of Health considers the telephone a luxury which cannot possibly be supplied by the local authority but offers the names and addresses of charities to which the very severely disabled might apply.'

A fifty-five-year-old couple in Yorkshire, the wife totally blind and in poor health, the man permanently incapacitated due to severe epilepsy from birth, were recommended by their doctor for a telephone. Both were confined to the house and lived on State supplementary benefits. The man suffered from violent fits and his blind wife was unable to help him. But the local welfare department told them that they were not entitled to a phone.

A sixty-four-year-old widow whose daughter was disabled by polio and was unable even to feed herself, went to inquire at a South London welfare department about the help she might be entitled to under the Act. She was told she should not believe all she read in the newspapers or heard on the radio as the authority had no money.

As unrest grew about the operation of the Act, Sir Keith Joseph told a deputation from the Disablement Income Group, in November 1970, that he aimed to evolve a strategy for the disabled and he offered to tell the organization some of his conclusions the following summer.

The next month a *Sunday Times* inquiry by Wendy Hughes revealed that many disabled people did not know whether they were registered or not. Field work by the Disablement Income Group and the Central Council for the Disabled had shown that 3.5 per cent of the population were disabled under the terms of the Morris Act. The true number of disabled was estimated to be around two million, whereas only 235,000 people were registered with local authorities. That is why Alfred Morris had argued in Parliament that there were well over one million missing from the register.

The *Sunday Times* had carried out a random survey of seventeen local authorities and this revealed that the number registered fell well below the figures one would expect from the estimated national average. This was the picture which emerged of the disabled registered as a percentage of the population of the various areas:

Hull, 1·21; Hounslow, 0·98; Kensington and Chelsea, 0·80; Rotherham, 0·70; Waltham Forest, 0·67; Plymouth, 0·60; Manchester, 0·58; Tower Hamlets, 0·53; Cardiff, 0·50; Bromley, 0·49; Bournemouth, 0·47; York, 0·42; Brent, 0·41; Gateshead, 0·40; Ipswich, 0·33; Coventry,

0·19. Coventry, in fact, with a population of 333,000 had only 645 registered disabled.

There can be no doubt that one reason why people were not coming forward to be registered was the lack of knowledge of the benefits that could follow. The Government had provided no official publicity about the Act. Although Whitehall had spent £60,000 in publicizing the new pensions for the over-eighties – the first reform to be introduced by the new Tory Government – nothing had been spent on official publicity about the Morris Act. It was estimated that only 100,000 people were affected by the pensions for over eighties, whereas some two million stood to benefit from the Morris reforms. The Government's failure to publicise the Act was made even more shameful by the fact that it had become a 'best seller' for Her Majesty's Stationery Office and was making a nice profit for the Exchequer.

On 18 December an indignant David Weitzman initiated a Commons debate on the implementation of the Act. He complained that three months after important sections of the measure had come into force, there was still remarkable ignorance of its provisions. Arthur Latham, Labour M.P. for Paddington North, gave details of local authorities that were denying knowledge of the Act.

Latham said that a social security officer in Exeter had denied to a woman that the Act had become law. A county council – Glamorgan – had sought to shelter behind the lack of a date for implementing Section (1) in order to postpone implementing Section (2).

Lewis Carter-Jones declared bitterly that while there was no division when the Bill was passing through Parliament, division was now creeping in as a result of the dilatory behaviour of Whitehall departments. The cause of sharpest division was the Government's refusal to take action to get a complete register of all the disabled. Michael Alison, Under Secretary for Health, again argued the astonishing case that the cost would be so great a diversion of resources – especially of manpower – that the whole point of the operation would be nullified. He insisted that there would be nothing left to meet the needs of the registered disabled.

Demand for services, he said, could be measured with a fair degree of accuracy by sampling and survey techniques. Lewis Carter-Jones interjected: 'A sample will never identify the people. Section One is about people.'

Alfred Morris declared that implementation of Section (1) was needed because it concerned a deeply serious human problem. It had to do with some of the poorest and most needy people as well as with preventable suffering.

Some of that preventable suffering concerned boys with muscular dystrophy whose parents were unaware even of the availability of ripple cushions. And because of this such boys were suffering serious and painful pressure sores.

In Hackney, twenty handicapped teenagers, mostly in wheelchairs, went out into the streets in January 1971 to test how easy it would be for them to get into public buildings. This follow-up to the Act – especially its provisions on access – was organised by Community Service volunteers. The disabled youngsters not only found steps barring their way to libraries, stations, lavatories and police stations, they found to their dismay that many officials were very unco-operative. The Act's message was clearly not getting through. Jack Ashley followed up early in February by leading a deputation of M.P.s to Sir Keith Joseph to demand that Section (1) should be put into operation without further delay.

A few days later Westminster, the wealthiest council in Britain, was obliged to call a press conference to defend itself against charges that it was neglecting disabled people in the Paddington area. Officials agreed that their register of 2,600 disabled – only about one per cent of the local population – was incomplete. Dr J. Briscoe-Smith, the Medical Officer of Health, confessed, too, that he was not proud of the council's record in the case of a woman who was still living in a damp room that had been reported eight months earlier.

The rumbling row over implementing the Act took a more serious turn on 27 February, when Alf Morris made a bitter public accusation that some local authorities were planning to deprive the disabled of their new deal. Angrily he declared: 'A document has come into my hands that prompts me to warn these authorities to stop tampering with the law.' He was referring to a memorandum prepared by the County Councils Association and the Association of Municipal Corporations. This interpreted in a mean-spirited manner the provision that authorities had a duty to provide and pay for telephones and television sets. Under the plan spelt out in the draft a disabled person would have to prove many things to become eligible for assistance. He would have to prove that he was unable to leave his house; was at risk when living alone or unaccompanied; was physically and mentally capable of using the instrument; was unable to afford to pay reasonable costs himself; and could not reasonably ask relatives to do so. Morris described the document as 'a most shocking and disturbing manoeuvre.' The criteria bore no relation to Parliament's intention. 'They are a hard-faced and cynical blue-print for diluting and evading the purpose of the law.' Morris warned: 'Any county council now considering the plan must be left in no doubt that it is both inexcusable and intolerable. It will be strenuously and implacably opposed.'

Evidence continued to build up of the determination of some authorities to evade their responsibilities. One councillor in Solihull accused that authority of stalling. He alleged that the council was being secretive because the provisions of the Act would push up the rates. There were some 3,000 disabled people in the area, but the council had not yet publicised the Act's provisions although it was nine months since it had become law.

Local authorities, far from being spurred into action, were given a further breathing space by the Government in February. Two months before David Weitzman had asked Sir Keith Joseph when he intended to implement Section (1) He was told that an announcement about the Order to bring this key section into operation would be made shortly after 1 April. He naturally assumed that the provisions of that section would be put into effect around that date. But in February the Health Department announced that soon after 1 April an Order would be made bringing the registration section into effect on 1 October.

The news came as a deep disappointment to Morris,

Ashley, Weitzman and their friends. It meant that thirteen months would have elapsed between the Act becoming law and this important section being made compulsory. They saw it as a clear invitation to the go-slow authorities to do nothing. Their measure still remained an Act mostly without action. The anniversary of the Bill's Third Reading in the Commons passed in March without celebration. The Commons campaigners saw no prospect of bridging the gap between good and bad authorities until the registration section came into effect and until authorities were instructed to seek out the disabled. The gap was the difference between a good authority like Kingston-upon-Hull which had already discovered twelve disabled people per thousand, and an authority like Canterbury that had managed to register only two per thousand. It was the difference between Oldham spending £70.83p per disabled person, and the Isle of Wight spending only 77p.

The British Polio Fellowship decided to do a spot check on how authorities were operating the new laws. They picked at random an authority in Greater London and took along a disabled member in a wheelchair to apply for help. They drove up to the office situated in a busy street where parking was prohibited. The entrance hall to the offices was cold, bleak and dirty. The lift was out of order, and it was too narrow for a wheelchair in any case. There was no inquiry desk on the ground floor and it was found two flights up. The official handling inquiries was told that there was a disabled person in a wheelchair on the ground floor requiring assistance. Fifteen minutes later another official arrived and without any apology for delay or attempt at a preamble fired off the usual type of questions. Name? Address? Are you known to anyone? What do you want? The disabled man explained that he needed some minor adaptations to his house. There were two awkward steps outside the house and one down to the bathroom that made life difficult for a person in a wheelchair. The official promised to send a social worker to inspect the premises but made no inquiry about when this would be convenient. As for knowing whether a telephone or T.V. was available under the Morris Act the official shook his head. He had no idea. These were only permissive recommendations, he misleadingly explained, so councils could act on them or not as they liked.

In fact, in the opinion of a number of local authorities the Act did not require them to do anything more than the previous permissive legislation. To be fair to authorities the Act had also reached the Statute Book at a difficult time for them. Not only were they short of money and staff, they were also involved in a major re-organization of their Social Service functions. The old separate departments which had handled mental health, child care, day nurseries and home helps were being merged into one Social Services Department. Moreover, in March 1971, the Government added more problems for the town and county halls by producing plans for a major re-organization of local government.

But critics of the local authorities and Government were given fresh ammunition in May with the publication of a massive survey on the handicapped and impaired. It was, in fact, a Government survey put in hand by the Wilson administration and carried out by Amelia Harris, Elizabeth Cox, Christopher Smith and Judith Buckle. The survey revealed that there were over three million people over sixteen living in private households in Britain who were suffering from some impairment. About one and a quarter million were men and one and three quarter million women. Almost half the men who had some impairment were aged sixty-five or over as were two thirds of the women. The survey gave this breakdown:

Very seriously handicapped, needing special care: 157,000; Severely handicapped, needing some support, 356,000; Appreciably handicapped, needing some support, 616,000; Impaired but needing little or no support, 1,942,000.

George Wilson, deputy director of the Central Council for the Disabled, commented: 'We have the facts; now it's time that local authorities and voluntary organizations got together to work out how to find the disabled, what their priorities for service should be, what the needs of the handicapped are, and how resources can be used to best advantage.'

A week before the anniversary of the Morris Act reaching the Statute Book Lewis Carter-Jones initiated a Friday Private Member's Debate in the Commons calling on the Government and local authorities to ensure full implementation of the measure. He opened by asserting: 'It would not be an exaggeration to say that progress has been abysmally slow.'

He argued that the Government's survey had revealed that the problem was more severe than M.P.s had realized when they were debating the Bill a year before. A major problem in making progress was that Government departments always thought in terms of cost. But Carter-Jones insisted that if cost-benefit analysis were applied properly it would be clear that the total cost of taking care of the disabled was far lower than had been made out. Another reason given for not implementing the Act was the re-organization of the welfare services into the Social Service Departments. Commented Carter-Jones: 'It is like saying we cannot send the lifeboat out to save people because we are painting it this week.'

He went on to make the point that if a local authority was asked to provide a ramp for a disabled person to enable him to get out of his home and refused to do so then it was guilty of imprisoning that person without trial.

Carter-Jones cited two cases to illustrate the ungenerous attitude being adopted by some authorities. Case one: A mother with a mentally handicapped girl of nineteen and a spastic girl of fourteen had a problem because the younger child could not get out of the house. The Warrington local authority had offered to put in a ramp but had said it would cost £45. The woman's husband had been unemployed for eleven months after breaking his leg in seven places; he had only just returned to work. Yet the authority concerned insisted on imposing the burden of that heavy bill on the family.

Case two: A severely disabled man in Huddersfield had a POSSUM unit provided by the Department of Health and was anxious to take a degree in English. But to carry

out his studies he needed a radio. The POSSUM unit had
an interface to take a radio but the local authority had
refused to provide one for what, on the face of it, seemed
a good reason: the man already had a radio. But he could
not operate that radio because he was paralysed. He could
only use a radio for his studies if it was the type that could be
fitted on the POSSUM unit.

Jack Ashley revealed that youth leaders in Stoke-on-Trent
had assured him they could compile a 100 per cent register of
disabled in the constituency in less than six months. But the
Government's unconstructive answer to that wonderful offer
had been that there would be considerable problems in using
voluntary effort, for instance, in giving the volunteers guidance to ensure an accurate assessment. The Government
also argued that each disabled person identified would have
to be visited afterwards by someone from the Social Services
Department and that because of the shortage of skilled
social workers this would involve watering-down what was
already being done for disabled people already registered.
Finally, the Government said that to register people would
raise false hopes. Commented Ashley: 'Hopes have already
been raised by the Act.'

Sir Keith Joseph began his reply to the debate by asserting
that the lessons of humanity and cost benefit both preached
the same doctrine: that the ideal to be aimed at was to keep
people at work, whether paid work or housework, and to keep
people at home. But when it came to registering people, he
insisted that there should be no compulsion. Alfred Morris,
however, had always stressed that registration should be
subject to the two essential principles of confidentiality and
voluntaryism. Sir Keith added that some people would not
want to be labelled, especially the mentally ill. The Government, nevertheless, was disturbed to learn from the survey
that there were 8,200 people in the most severely disabled
categories living alone – 8,000 of them women, mostly old.
It was thought that probably 6,000 of them received local
authority services but he wanted local authorities to search
out these people and ensure that they had all the help they
needed.

As an immediate practical step Sir Keith revealed that he had decided to assist disabled people who were not within easy reach of a lavatory at home. He had decided that local authorities should be asked to carry out research with chemical closets now being produced for the growing caravan industry. He proposed to buy 1,000 such closets immediately for this operation.

This announcement was to bring an astonished reaction in the House of Lords a few days later from Baroness Summerskill. She asserted that progressive local authorities had been providing such chemical closets for years. She challenged the need for any more research to prove their usefulness. The Lords were also debating the implementation of the Act. Lord Longford described it as perhaps the greatest single legislative achievement of a Private Member that any of them could remember. This was no small tribute.

Lady Masham said the proposal that telephones should be provided had caused more controversy than any other section. She cited the case of a North Riding authority that had refused to supply a telephone to two very severely disabled people living alone, one virtually immobile. Their doctor had said a phone would be a safety link and was justifiable as a possible means of saving life.

Lord Wells-Pestell, chairman of a national voluntary organization, had first-hand knowledge of the tight-fisted attitude of some authorities. His organization, which had been providing radio and T.V. to bedridden, house-bound and old people for over thirty years, had been inundated with requests from such local authorities seeking free radio and television sets to pass on to disabled people. In the course of conservation several officials had said that their authorities had no intention of implementing Section (2) of the Act, dealing with the provision of a wide range of services and equipment.

Lord Cullen of Ashbourne had sat in the Lords for thirty-nine years without making a speech. He ended his long silence with a helpful maiden speech in this debate. As a financier his opinion that a relatively small outlay of rate-payers' money to assist the disabled to live at home could save a much larger cost for hospital treatment was particularly useful. Lack of money was a major reason for failure to provide facilities listed in the Act. Sir Keith Joseph, questioned on this problem in the Commons, replied in May that the Financial Resolution passed by the Wilson Government was not a commitment to increase spending but merely an authority to do so.

Behind the scenes there had been sharp exchanges involving Shadow Chancellor Roy Jenkins and Sir Keith. Jenkins wrote to Sir Keith on 4 May strongly challenging a statement made by him the previous month that the Act 'carried with it no finance whatsoever' and 'had no finance connected with it'. He recalled that the Labour Government had approved a Money Resolution covering the Bill. 'If this had not been done' wrote Jenkins, 'the Bill could not have made progress, although it was not at that stage necessary to make any precise estimate of its cost.' Jenkins also pointed out that the Bill did not receive Royal Assent until the final day of the last Parliament. This point was made because it explained why the Labour Government had been unable to follow up the Money Resolution with an announcement of the sum of money to be allocated to the new Act. Jenkins angrily accused Sir Keith of misleading the House of Commons. He complained that it did not help for the 'utterly inaccurate impression' to be given that it was an Act which had somehow reached the Statute Book without any provisions being made for money to pay for it. What particularly angered Alfred Morris and his friends was that the Government's attitude was encouraging those local authorities who were not anxious to act and were using lack of finance as an excuse.

Sir Keith, however, stuck by his argument that the Money Resolution was not a commitment to increase expenditure. He was sheltering behind a technicality. He was certainly not acting in the spirit of the move by Tory leaders just before the General Election, when Lord Balniel pledged on their behalf that if the Morris Bill were lost the next Conservative Government would introduce a similar measure. The Tory Shadow Cabinet members who approved that vote-winning statement were well aware that the Act would require money to make some of its most important provisions effective. They had not gone so far as to pledge financial provision 'at a stroke' – but morally they were committed up to the hilt.

~~~~~~

Chapter Eleven

Breakthrough

DISAPPOINTMENT there had been in no small measure in the year that had passed since the Morris Act reached the Statute Book. But the picture was by no means one of unrelieved gloom. Moreover, it was getting a little brighter with every month that passed. By mid-1971, it was becoming very clear that the Act had already succeeded in creating a new public awareness of the problems and needs of disabled and chronically sick people. Certain newspapers, both national and local, had set themselves up as watchdogs and were continually highlighting the shortcomings of those local authorities who were slow in implementing the measure.

Finance was still a major problem and looked like remaining so for as far ahead as anyone could see. But the Government had made provision for an initial increase of twelve per cent in local authority spending on services for the handicapped in 1971-72, which was to be doubled in 1972-73. This spending helped Section (2) of the Morris Act – the section requiring local authorities to provide a wide range of services for the handicapped, ranging from telephones to adaptations to homes. In addition the spending of £3 million was announced for the purposes of Section (17) of the Act – the building of special hospital units, away from geriatric wards, for the young chronic sick.

Another £12 million a year had been committed by Sir Keith for payment from December 1971 of a new attendance allowance to help in cases where severely disabled people had to be cared for by their families. The allowance of £4·80p a week was expected to be paid to some 50,000 or more. To qualify, the physically or mentally disabled had to require attention both during the day and night. The allowance was to be tax free and paid irrespective of means. A proposal for such an attendance allowance had first appeared in an early draft of the Morris Bill and had been included in the Wilson Government's National Superannuation Bill which had not reached the Statute Book. Sir Keith had also taken up another proposal abandoned by the Wilson Government in its ill-judged rush to the polls – an improved earnings rule for the working wives of the chronic sick. As Sir Keith acknowledged, this proposal had also made its legislative debut in an early draft of the Morris Bill.

A new invalidity allowance for the chronic sick was being brought in, too. This was to be on a less ambitious basis than one proposed by the Wilson government but it was to be introduced much earlier.

A higher insurance benefit for the dependent children of the chronic sick – a new proposal of Sir Keith's – was also to be introduced by the end of the year.

On his general strategy for the disabled, Sir Keith spelt out his thoughts at a meeting of the Disablement Income Group in June 1971. It was an important speech, although it did not contain a list of dramatic new proposals, and it showed that the ground was being prepared for advances on a number of fronts.

On the important question of work, he revealed that the Department of Employment had started a comprehensive internal inquiry into their policies on employment for the disabled. The investigation included a review of the situation in Remploy factories and sheltered workshops run by local authorities and voluntary bodies.

On the future, Sir Keith had something to say about the possibility of some type of invalidity pension. If money were available the Government might provide some form of benefit for the disabled which was not means-tested and yet was not contributory either. This would be of particular interest to those who had to rely on supplementary benefit.

But though the Government knew roughly the field where it would like to help, ministers still needed to know a great deal more about how the people concerned lived – what kind of improvement would be most welcome to the family caring for them and to the disabled person himself. Sir Keith said this department was considering setting up a research survey into the circumstances of people of working age who were absent from work because of medium or long term periods of sickness or disability.

Sir Keith had not announced any new departure but it was clear from his words that a log jam was moving in Whitehall—one jammed for too long by complacency, apathy and ignorance. The relentless pressure of the voluntary agencies working on public opinion and Whitehall had done much to bring this about. But the publicity given to the Morris Act was probably the biggest single factor that had stirred the interest as well as the conscience of the public. It had made the plight of the disabled a major public talking point at last.

This breakthrough was confirmed by the fact that after years of neglect the two main parties decided to debate the subject at their annual conferences in the autumn of 1971.

Tory rank-and-file speakers showed a lively awareness of the problems of the disabled and were far from satisfied with the action taken in the previous few years. Opening a debate on Social Security and Health, Alderman Mrs Ann Spokes of Oxford paid tribute to the fact that one of the first Acts passed by the Heath Government had provided an attendance allowance for the severely disabled – but she stressed that as with most new schemes there were anomalies.

She hoped it would be possible to be more generous and to adopt a less strict interpretation of need, especially where badly disabled children were concerned. She urged that the next step should be a national disability allowance which recognized the extra expense incurred by the disabled, including those who were helping themselves in full-time jobs.

Lady Chetwynd, from Berkshire, told the conference that voluntary workers could do a useful job in identifying need. The only certain way of finding the handicapped was to do a house-to-house survey – in fact, the type of operation that had been envisaged by the Morris Act.

Sir Keith Joseph, faced with the impatient demands of delegates conceded: 'There is a huge amount to be done.' He added significantly: 'Perhaps the biggest task still ahead of us is in connection with the disabled.'

There was a significant contribution, too, at the Labour Party conference debate on the need to implement the Morris Act. It came from Jack Ashley M.P., and it cut through whatever temptation there might have been for political posturing and humbug. He pointed out that while Labour Party members condemned the Tories for providing an inadequate constant attendance allowance, they should remember that some ministers in the last Labour Government had made exactly the same kind of speeches about the cost of such an allowance. 'So our Government, better as it was than the Conservatives, was not good enough in its attitude to the disabled; and we really require a comprehensive policy to be planned for the future.'

Another speaker pointed out that the Transport Workers' Union was one of the employers not taking up its quota of three per cent disabled.

There could not be so much talk by the rank-and-file politicians without some progress at ground level, too. The picture in the autumn of 1971 may not have been cause for general congratulation. But neither was it one of unrelieved gloom. It was still easy to find local authorities in whose areas the Act had made little or no impact. But there was a growing number of other authorities with a good record of activity and achievement. The number of disabled registered with Liverpool Corporation had risen from 4,700 to 11,000 during the year. This dramatic increase had followed a leaflet distribution to all 220,000 households in the city. Expenditure on the handicapped was estimated to be already £25,000 up on the same period for the previous year. The number of registered disabled in Manchester had increased by some

1,800 during the short life-time of the Act and new cases were being added at the rate of 5,000 a year. Over 400 free telephones had also been provided by that corporation alone, and more than 270 properties had been adapted since April. By May, 1972, more than 1,000 telephones had been installed. Similarly remarkable but little-publicized progress had been made by local authorities in many widely differing parts of Britain. Dr Brian Meredith Davies, Director of Social Services for Liverpool, expressed the belief that the Morris Act had produced a momentum which it is hard to achieve in local government. Even Salford, on the black list of low spenders on the disabled, had got as far as distributing 4,500 leaflets in an effort to trace those in need.

In London two thirds of the boroughs had taken action. One of the most imaginative efforts to track down the needy had been made by Hackney. There the borough council had organized a motorcade through the streets on a Saturday morning, had issued 25,000 leaflets, and organized a visit by disc jockey Jimmy Saville to help publicize the survey. This borough, one of the poorest in London, had also paid for the installation of 130 telephones in 1971. It had estimated that if every London borough were to contribute only £120 each they could pay for a thirty second television commercial at a peak viewing time. The idea, however, was not taken up. Some boroughs admitted that such an advert could cause an explosion in demand that they simply could not meet. Could not – or would not? Ten London boroughs, in fact, had done nothing about implementing Section (1) of the Act. They were Barking, Bexley, Croydon, Enfield, Newham, Redbridge, Richmond, Southwark, Waltham Forest and Wandsworth. The laggards were spotlighted by Des Wilson in a survey in the London *Evening Standard* designed to shame them into action.

Such was the interest in the problem by the autumn of 1971 that any authority dragging its feet was likely to be publicly exposed. Take Birmingham, for instance: this great authority had decided to do things on the cheap by providing house-bound, and even dangerously isolated, invalids with whistles rather than phones with which to summon help in emergencies. One such whistle was provided for Mrs Ann Price, a thirty-seven-year-old housewife, confined to a wheelchair because of multiple sclerosis. She was alone all day while her husband was at work and her fourteen-year-old son was at school. Mrs Price tried blowing her whistle without effect. Local Labour M.P. Mr Denis Howell was called in to put it to the test. He was a good choice – in fact a very experienced whistle-blower as he had been a Football League referee. But not even Mr Howell could attract any attention. The exercise, however, had attracted the attention of the national press. As Birmingham blushed, Mr Howell explained to reporters: 'I blew as hard as I would in front of a crowd of 60,000. All that happened was that a man got out of his car and listened before driving away.'

It is unlikely that, if an authority had thought of providing a disabled person with a whistle a few years earlier, such an incident would have aroused indignation or the interest of the newspapers.

Another sign of progress came from Cardiff. The city council, despite the fact that it was busily engaged in fighting a major battle against the Government's plan to demote the city to a district council and put it under the thumb of Glamorgan county, sponsored a one-day conference on planning for the disabled. The inspiration for the conference had come from Ewart Parkinson, Director of Planning for the city. Parkinson, a man of considerable vision, had been responsible for introducing Professor Colin Buchanan to Cardiff to replan the city centre, but he admits that up to 1971 he had not given a great deal of thought to the problems of planning for handicapped people. Such a conference two years earlier would have attracted no more than about a hundred people. But such was the awareness that had been aroused that over five hundred applied to attend and several hundred had to be turned away.

A useful filip to registration was given in November by *Which*, the magazine of the Consumer Association. It produced a report which showed that handicapped people who were not registered were not getting the help they needed.

Those who were registered were, on the whole, getting aids and services. The report was based on interviews with 110 physically handicapped people in the previous twelve months in Reading and the London Borough of Wandsworth.

One case in the survey was of Mrs H., aged sixty-six, suffering from osteo-arthritis in both legs. She had considerable difficulty getting around and relied on a lot of help from her husband, who was only on light work himself as the result of a coronary. She needed a raised lavatory seat, aids to help her dress and a pick-up stick. But she did not know she could get them through her local authority or hospital. She was attending a hospital out-patients' clinic but said no one had ever asked her how she managed at home or suggested that the local authority Social Services Department was there to help.

Two-thirds of those interviewed were not registered with their local Social Services Department, nor were they known to the Health Department. Some seemed to feel there might be a social stigma attached in going to the 'welfare'. This no doubt resulted from lack of the right type of publicity about the services available. *Which* concluded that the local authorities needed to spell out and publicize how they could help the handicapped.

Evidence continued to grow during the autumn of 1971 that, despite the initial disappointment about slow implementation, the Act had aroused a lively new interest in the problems of the disabled. In an increasing number of spheres that interest was being translated into action.

Post Office engineers throughout Wales decided in November to make their contribution by volunteering to work without pay to install telephones for those eligible to receive them under the Act. The scheme was the outcome of a new agreement between the Post Office Engineering Union and the Wales and Marches Telecommunications Board. Under this P.O.E.U. members agreed to install phones after normal working hours, during the evenings and at weekends. The Wales Board agreed to make vehicles and materials available. The Post Office also agreed to cut the charge of connection by half. The *Daily Express* in a congratulatory leader described the engineers' gesture as warming and thoughtful, but it urged the Post Office to go the whole way and scrap the connection fee. Declared the newspaper: 'Let generosity be full-hearted.'

Lord Delacourt-Smith, general secretary of the P.O.E.U., congratulated the Welsh members for 'their noble public service gesture'. He hoped local councils would regard this initiative as a means of doubling the number of telephones installed under the Act rather than reducing the overall expenditure. Mr Vic Feather, T.U.C. General Secretary, applauded the move and commented: 'It fits remarkably into the spirit of the campaign we are now running to relieve the elderly – the pensioners – from loneliness and poverty.'

Evidence of an effort by Monmouthshire to get to grips with the problem of access to places of entertainment came at about the same time. A new entertainment centre to contain cinemas and bingo halls was to be built at Cwmbran, and a year or two before no attention would have been paid to the fact that handicapped people would be barred from using the facilities because the centre was sited on an upper floor with no lifts. But now that the Act was law the Monmouthshire planning authority tackled the developers about the problem of access for disabled people. Local newspapers reported the affair and a county spokesman was reported as saying: 'Not to have done so (tackled the developer) would have gone against all we believe in.' The authority proposed to talk to the developer before confirming planning permission in an effort to improve the situation for the local disabled people.

In London even the laggard borough of Richmond decided that it was time to make some improvements to its social services following criticism by the press, television and national and voluntary organizations, which stemmed in part from the existence of the Act.

On the Whitehall front the Department of Health and Social Security produced the first of the annual reports on research and development of equipment for the disabled provided for under Section (22) of the Act. It announced that a fact-finding group had been set up in the ministry to investigate needs and recommend action. Among examples of work in progress, support was being given to a university engineering department for a project aimed at producing a step-climbing electrically powered wheelchair. The report was greeted as a modest start in a vast field. The aim of Section (22) had been to stimulate action to bring technology to the aid of severely disabled people. It looked as though future reports would reflect that priority.

But even as the new deal born of the Morris Act began to take shape on the ground the pressure groups stepped up their campaigns for more action. One such move came from the Association for Research into Restricted Growth, set up the previous year with the indefatigable Charles Pocock of the Disabled Drivers' Association as its national chairman. Baroness Phillips, president of the association, asked the first parliamentary question on its behalf in December 1971. She pressed the Government to consider strengthening the Morris Act so as to include specific reference to people of restricted growth. A few days before, television viewers had seen a film produced by Lord Snowdon called 'Born to be Small'. Lady Phillips told the Lords that any who had seen that film would have realized that people of small stature were not confined to the stage and circus but were carrying out all kinds of work. But the help which the small person could get depended at present on the sensitivity of individuals in the health and welfare areas. This was not satisfactory. The small person moved self-consciously in an unfriendly world of derision and in-dignity. The Government should amend the Act to help him. But the Government, through Lord Aberdare, Minister of State for Health, rejected the request as unnecessary on the ground that small people already had access to existing services.

Charles Pocock commented later: 'Under the Morris Act all the benefits should flow from Section One. We want local authorities to recognize that in preparing their registers under that section the person of small stature should be included. We want a directive sent from the Health Department to local authorities.'

On the general problem Pocock says: 'We want an understanding that people of small stature are ordinary people trying to use the talents they have – not peculiar people to be exploited in the circus. We want to get across that they have ambitions, desires and talents like any other people. One of our members, for instance, is a General Practitioner. He is four feet two inches. Society has exploited small stature in the past and we still suffer from this. There's a psychological barrier to break. There's also the problem of medical research into how to alleviate physical limitations. We want children who suffer from small stature to be treated as normal boys and girls and given normal educational opportunities.'

Pocock's association judges that there are about 3,000 people of small stature in Britain – a thousand more than the Government estimate. The problem is to get them to come forward.

For some months there had been rumblings of complaint about the application of Sir Keith Joseph's new weekly attendance allowance, due to come into operation in December 1971. The allowance, a standard £4·80p was to be paid to adults of any age over sixteen, and under separate rules for children aged two to sixteen. Need for attendance had to be proved and one of two tests satisfied. For six months before the allowance is payable the disabled person must have been so severely afflicted either physically or mentally that he requires frequent attention from another person throughout the day and prolonged or repeated attention throughout the night. Alternatively he must require continual supervision in order to avoid substantial danger to himself or others. For a disabled child it is also necessary to prove that his need for attention is more than the normal requirements of a child of that age.

Sir Keith told the Commons shortly before the new allowance was to be paid out that at least 44,000 severely disabled people, many of them cared for by their families, would benefit. His target of 50,000 was within reach and would eventually be exceeded. Sir Keith went on to say that 95,000 claims had been received up to 23 November, of

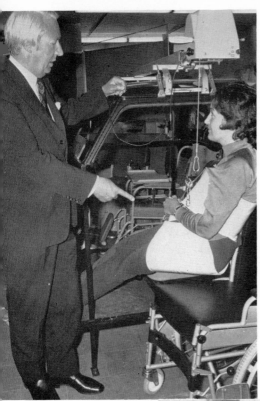

Prime Minister Mr Edward Heath operates a hoist during his visit to the Living Foundation's Aids Centre, Kensington High Street, in 1971.

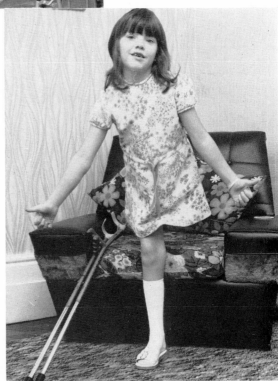

...linda was eight when they ...moved her leg. She says, 'It's ...en blown away by the wind.'
...otograph by courtesy of the 'Hornsey ...rnal'.

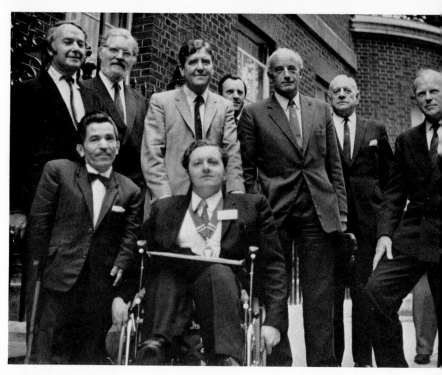

A deputation of leading campaigners for disabled drivers calls at No. 10 Downing Street to p̣
their case to Prime Minister Edward Heath.

Back (*left to right*) James Loring (Spastics Society), Duncan Guthrie (Central Council for t̩
Disabled), Alfred Morris, M.P., Donald Powell (Secretary British Polio Foundation), N̩
Marten, M.P., Commander Radford (British School of Motoring), Monty Woodhouse, M.P.

Front (*left to right*) Charles Pocock (Secretary Disabled Drivers' Association), Joseph Hennes̩
(Chairman, Disabled Drivers' Association).

Reproduced by courtesy of the Disabled Drivers' Association.

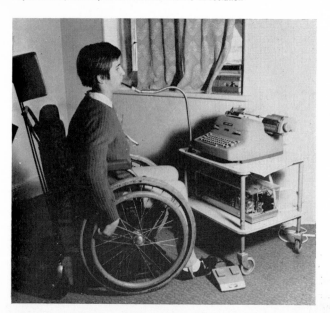

Possum at work. Ma̩
Older, a severely hand̩
capped spastic, blov̩
down a tube to use h̩
patient-operated select̩
mechanisms (Possur̩
typewriter.

which 30,000 were still being considered by the Attendance Allowance Board, which had the difficult task of deciding which cases qualified. Sir Keith declared: 'It is a highly satisfactory outcome, so far.' Opinion on that point was far from unanimous. Some welfare workers had been outraged by some of the harrowing cases turned down by the Board. They complained bitterly that the tests applied to cases were far too strict. As the new allowance came into operation the Disablement Income Group launched a strong attack on the set-up. It pointed out that thousands of severely disabled people were disqualified from claiming the allowance because they could sleep at night. Sometimes they slept only with the help of sedatives. Many had spent considerable sums on special beds and heating equipment in order to rest properly. After studying several hundred applications the group had decided that the criteria must be amended. It cited the following cases in support of its campaign:

Case 1: A Mr W. who had suffered from muscular dystrophy for twenty-five years had not qualified because he could not satisfy the condition of needing prolonged or repeated attention during the night. Yet it was agreed by the Board's review doctor and the disabled man's own doctor that he could not be left alone for more than half an hour and could not manage without assistance to get out of bed, walk, dress, or go to the lavatory. The doctors also agreed that Mr W. could not even change position in bed at night without help, but that as he used a mechanical bed he did not have to be moved periodically to avoid pressure sores or discomfort. He was therefore disqualified for an attendance allowance.

Case 2: Mrs T., aged thirty-three, a spastic with a four-month old baby, had been ruled out because she did not meet the alternative condition of needing continual supervision to avoid substantial danger. But she often bumped into furniture and if she fell out of her wheelchair she could not get back again. Both the board's doctor and her own agreed that she required someone during the night and day.

The group believed that another 100,000 adults and 25,000 children should be brought within the scope of the scheme.

Mr Stuart Lyon, a group official, said the aim was to have the benefit awarded to people needing attention day and night. After that they wanted to see the introduction of a national disability income to help cover such extra expenses as special equipment, special diets and extra wear and tear on clothes.

Another pressure group for the disabled took action in November 1971, to persuade Parliament to legislate on their behalf. The Kidney Research Unit for Wales Foundation under the chairmanship of Max Gabe-Wilkinson, a dynamic Cardiff businessman, launched a petition to urge Parliament to pass legislation to facilitate the speedy transplantation of kidneys from dead people to those whose kidneys were diseased. It was launched in the light of the grim fact that over 7,000 people die of kidney disease each year in Britain. Gabe-Wilkinson explained to a Cardiff press conference that because kidneys deteriorate very rapidly and must be removed within an hour of death there was a very real need to enable doctors to act swiftly, while protecting the rights and dignity of the individual. He believed this could be accomplished by a Bill to permit the removal of the kidneys from a person certified dead by at least two independent doctors unless the person had objected in writing during his lifetime to the removal of his organs. The move stirred up a lively controversy in view of its attempt to persuade Parliament to accept the principle of 'opting out'.

Meanwhile M.P.s got down to legislating on another issue affecting the disabled – the 'rackets' operated by certain firms claiming to help the handicapped. This scandal had been raised during debates on the Alf Morris Bill, and in January 1972 Mr David Reed, Labour M.P. for Sedgefield, got a second reading for a Bill he had introduced to deal with it. It sought to make certain that only charitable organizations would be able to claim through door-to-door salesmen that what they were doing was on behalf of the disabled. Reed had the support of M.P.s of all parties in attacking firms who employed disabled people for small wages and then used salesmen to sell shoddy goods on the doorstep and made high profits by claiming that the proceeds went to help the handicapped.

By the end of 1971 the adverse publicity for areas with bad records on the registration of disabled people and spending on services had become so embarrassing that the Government decided not to release any more figures. Sir Keith Joseph refused a Commons request for such information from Jack Ashley, M.P. Ashley tackled the Prime Minister. Mr Heath replied that there was no question of concealing information of public importance, and he defended Sir Keith's decision on the ground that the figures released on previous occasions had been used to draw unwarranted conclusions about the activities of local authorities. The government may have been influenced by the experience of such authorities as Canterbury which had been shown to have one of the worst records in the country. The local Labour Party had campaigned strongly on this issue in the local elections and the Conservatives had lost power in that city for the first time for many years. It was becoming increasingly unsafe for any local council to neglect the needs of the handicapped.

The Government itself had taken note of the new public interest and had quietly changed the tone of its guidance to local authorities on the issue of identification and registration. In a circular of September 1971, which followed up the much criticized circular of August 1970, it told local authorities that they would be faced with the ultimate task of identifying everyone who had needs and wanted a service. It added: 'The completion of this task should in any case be the authority's aim . . ."

Duncan Guthrie, looking back over the first eighteen months of the Morris Act, expressed the belief in January 1972 that it had made a great contribution. 'It has produced a wonderful change in the position of the disabled. As a result of the great publicity it has attracted public attitudes have changed.'

But Guthrie thought there was still too much latitude for local authorities. 'They have to satisfy themselves that there is a need. They are judge and jury in their own case.'

He hoped that all authorities would work within the spirit as well as the wording of the Act. Most important of all was the attitude to be adopted towards the disabled in the future. A disabled person should not be embarrassed by his disability. 'He is just an ordinary person who has a disability just as I have a beard.'

In April, 1972, two developments clearly underlined the effectiveness of the Morris Act.

The Isle of Wight which, as a result of the Act, had carried out a survey of the chronically sick and disabled, discovered that there were 3,000 such people on the island—not 600 as had previously been assumed. The island, which had been criticized for not spending enough on Social Services, was the first County to carry out such a house to house survey to track down the crippled.

In the Commons Dr Dickson Mabon, Labour and Co-op M.P. for Greenock, introduced a Bill to extend to Scotland all the provisions of sections 1 and 2 of the Act. He did so following a report in the *British Medical Journal* by Ralph and Gillian Johnson which warned that Scotland's exclusion from those sections might cause her to fall further behind England. The article revealed that there had been no apparent attempt by local authorities to identify the disabled, as was required in England.

Afterword

∿∿∿∿∿∿∿∿∿∿∿∿∿∿∿∿∿∿∿∿

by Alfred Morris

I T W A S A complaint of some of Sir Edwin Chadwick's supporters in the battle to implement the Public Health Act 1848 that they had no real opposition. By this they meant that their opponents were never really frank. Of course, the Act had no shortage of opponents. They included anti-interventionists, critics of centralization, obscurantists, nit-pickers and others who, like John Bright and the affluent slum and chimney owners, had important vested interests to defend. Also among them were the fat but filthy local worthies of *Cess-cum-Poolton* from Dickens's biting satire. Sir Edwin Chadwick's supporters came to be known as the 'clean' party. But few of his opponents liked Lord Palmerston's attempt to lump them altogether as the 'dirty' party. Their public criticisms of the Act rarely reflected their private reasons for opposing its implementation. Instead, they dressed up their motives in pretty, if grandiose, talk of local freedom and the red-blooded Englishman's rights.

The more things change, as the Frenchman says, the more they remain the same. I have often been reminded of Lord Palmerston's taunt about the 'clean' and 'dirty' parties by those who have tried, since the Royal Assent, to delay and obstruct the implementation of the Chronically Sick and Disabled Persons Act 1970. They disliked being thought of as opponents in principle of the new legislation. By comparison with the 'dirty' party, they were at once more furtive and faceless. They were at first not only unwilling to identify the disabled, but often reluctant even to identify themselves. They were not silver-tongued orators, but tight-lipped sabo-teurs. They eschewed public debate, in favour of snag-finding and the procedural ploy in committee. They liked to see themselves as shrewd local businessmen and dragged their feet as quietly as possible. But like the 'dirty' party, in many localities they have provided a strong opposition in the short-term. For this, as I hope to show, central government as well as the local snag-finders must accept responsibility.

The Act has been fully in force since 1 December 1971. It became law entirely without party animus and with the clear intention of Parliament that it would be implemented in the same atmosphere of co-operation. The size and gravity of the problems tackled by the Act are no longer in doubt. The Government's own survey has given the facts. They are worse even than I feared when I began to draft my Bill. The official survey – by the Office of Population Censuses and Surveys – excluded all disabled children and young people under the age of sixteen and also many handicapped people over the age of sixty-five. Nevertheless, the survey found that there are *three million* people lacking part or all of a limb, organism or mechanism of the body. Again excluding those under sixteen years of age and many elderly handicapped people, the survey revealed a figure of 1·28 *million* adults with much more serious handicaps, many of whom are house-bound and isolated without any kind of help. Our preliminary estimate of a 'missing million' from the local disablement registers is thus shown to have been a conserva-tive estimate by the Government's own published figures. Nor is there any question now of the validity of the concept of the disabled family. It is nowhere denied that there are millions of non-disabled people who, through family, are personally involved in the problems of severe disablement in Britain today. Indeed, it is increasingly accepted now that we can help many disabled people only if we are prepared to help the family as a whole.

As well as amending thirty-nine other Acts of Parliament, including such major statutes as the War Pensions Act 1921 the Public Health Act 1936, the Education Act 1944, the,

National Health Service Act 1946, the National Assistance Act 1948 and the Housing Act 1957, the new Act makes provisions in fields where previously there was no legislation of any kind to amend. These latter include the five sections of the Act on improving access and facilities for severely disabled people at public and social buildings. The most important of these affects new buildings or premises to which the public are to be admitted, *whether on payment or otherwise*. Section (8), which amends the Education Act 1944, as well as the Education (Scotland) Act 1962, specifically extends the new order to universities and other educational buildings. As we have seen, access to buildings is fundamentally important to improving the social status of many disabled people and their families. On grounds of cost, there was no prospect of our being able to enforce the adaptation of all *existing* buildings. There was, however, the expectation, on both sides of both Houses of Parliament, that existing buildings would be adapted, wherever possible, in the spirit of the Act. Full adaptation of existing buildings can be extremely difficult as well as costly. But minor adaptations, even of old buildings, is neither as difficult nor as costly as some would have us believe. The London borough of Haringey provides a good example of how to proceed. After carrying out a survey of all public buildings, the borough Council decided what adaptations were necessary and its access project was carefully costed. A full report of the survey was then made available to the Central Council for the Disabled and constructive discussion immediately took place on its implementation.

The important lead given by the authorities of the two Houses of Parliament, in making the Palace of Westminster accessible to disabled people and providing there the facilities they need, also deserves to be much more widely followed. Many more adaptations could and should be made to existing public and social buildings than have so far been attempted. That local access campaigns receive widespread public support has been amply demonstrated already. But there is still need for vigorous campaigning on this issue in localities throughout Britain. As well as insisting that the law is fully enforced in respect of new buildings, pressure for adaptations must now be intensified. If the disabled person is to be helped to live as normal a life as possible, we must also intensify pressure for improved access at places of work and to every kind of public transport.

Inevitably perhaps, most public attention has so far been directed to the response of local authorities to the new mandatory charter of local services for the long-term sick and disabled in Section (2) of the Act. This is the section which ensures the availability in every locality of practical assistance in the home, housing adaptations, television and radio, telephones and any special equipment necessary to enable the disabled person to use a telephone, educational and home library facilities, holidays, meals in the home or elsewhere, transport to and from local services outside the home, and many other forms of community help. It is impossible here to notice all that has been done by the 'good' local authorities since Section (2) came into force. Not only have its provisions been fully and humanely applied in many widely differing parts of Britain. It has now been proved beyond argument that all the purposes of the Act can be fully met, in current conditions, except perhaps to those whom Sir Edwin Chadwick would have accused of ' . . . giving to misery all they have to give – a sneer.'

Yet the 'good' local authorities have received much less publicity than the snag-finders. It is, for example, a much better known fact that Birmingham supplied whistles, for use by home-bound disabled people in emergencies, than that Manchester had already provided over 400 telephones for such people within a year of the Act receiving the Royal Assent. Again, it is less well known that Hackney, one of the poorest of the London boroughs, had paid for 130 telephones for disabled people at a time when well-publicised Richmond, one of the richest of the London boroughs, had installed only one. Even the unprecedented action of the Welsh members of the Post Office Engineering Union in contracting to install telephones under the Act in their own time, *and without pay*, appears to have received less publicity than Birmingham's whistles. Of disabled women, the report of the Government's own survey found that: ' . . . even one in twenty of those who need special care has no one living with her, having to bang on walls to attract the attention of neighbours, provided they are at home.' This was the position immediately before the Act came into force. There is no longer any justification for home-bound disabled people to be dangerously isolated in this way, or for the other serious deprivations detailed in the Government's report. As the 'good' local authorities have shown, it is also no longer even frank to argue that severely disabled people need be treated differently by different local authorities.

The Act's furtive opponents have not saved public money by failing to provide the new charter of local services for handicapped people. In fact, they have *wasted* public money. For the severely handicapped person who is not helped to live at home often has to be hospitalized, or otherwise institutionalized, at very much higher cost to public funds. This is now readily, if belatedly, conceded by central government. Whitehall has come to recognize that one of the best ways of easing the strain on the hospital service is to extend and improve domiciliary care, so that more and more severely handicapped people can live at home. Yet Ministers have been strangely loath to tell the local snag-finders and feet-draggers to get a move on in meeting their responsibilities under the Act. Those who suffer include needful disabled people who have no feet to drag. This is why the Act's supporters in some localities have been tempted to say that the alternative to getting on is getting out. They insist that local authority leaders who neither share, nor even want to understand, the philosophy of the Act will soon have to make way for those who do.

The most urgent and constructive step that ministers could now take is further to increase central government's stake in the cost of providing all the local services laid down by the Act. This would make for much more rapid nationwide implementation of all its provisions. There is no value in recognizing that improved home-care can ultimately help the taxpayer if ministers stubbornly refuse to allocate the resources necessary for the new local services to develop. It is self-defeating for central government to deny local councils money which they can spend not only with more humanity than Whitehall, but also with improved cost effectiveness. Since the Act became law, there have been two annual increases of twelve per cent in Whitehall's stake in local spending on the chronically sick and disabled. But the Government's own estimate of the size of the disablement problem itself provides eloquent testimony to the inadequacy of these increases. Moreover, they are unspecific increases which have been wrapped up in the total rate support grant from central to local government. In the words of the Secretary of State for Social Services, Sir Keith Joseph: '... local authority expenditure on social services for the chronically sick and disabled forms part of the total relevant expenditure attracting rate support grant ...'

Whether every local council has in fact spent the two annual increases on the chronically sick and disabled, for whom they were intended, is doubted even among expert observers. There is a pressing need now both for an increase in the amount, and a review of the method of allocating, Whitehall's stake in expenditure under the Act. It is undeniably in the public interest that central government should now opt for new-style grants of increased amount. We have had a plethora of well-intentioned words. But they are no substitute for well-judged action to allow much higher numbers of severely handicapped people to live in comfort and dignity in the community. If ministers want quickly to help in closing the gap between the 'good' and 'bad' local councils, as they claim to do, they must devise a special rate support grant for services provided under the Act. They will not close the gap by means of annual percentage increases, even if they are at a much higher level than the two so far agreed. The percentage increase tends to confirm, rather than reduce, local differences in standards of provision. The Act strongly insists on a high *general* standard of local authority services for the chronically sick and disabled. If financial arrangements ill-suited to this purpose continue to thwart its achievement it will be no excuse for ministers to argue that they were defeated by procedure. Bold and imaginative leadership is required to defeat a major human and social problem. By unanimously approving the Money Resolution associated with my Bill, Parliament gave its undoubted sanction for any additional expenditure arising under the Act. This should have meant a much more generous allocation of resources from central to local government than has so far been given. The laggard local councils should already have been given a date by which their services for the chronically sick and disabled would have to be raised to the level intended by Parliament in enacting my Bill.

Nowhere is the cost of inadequate Exchequer support for local services seen more clearly than in the moribund and barrack-like buildings in which large numbers of mentally handicapped people are detained. As the Campaign for the Mentally Handicapped has affirmed, they are not so much hospitals as sad anti-hospitals. In a report from one hospital board, some of these institutions are described as 'perfect examples of human warehouses'. Ministers themselves have stated that as many as a half of their inmates could be set free, *if* local authority services can be improved. Whitehall admits that most of the inmates are not in need of continuous medical or nursing care, do not need 'assistance to feed, wash or dress' and even have 'no physical handicap or severe behaviour difficulties'. In a statement to the House of Commons, the Secretary of State for Social Services has stated: 'We stress the need to accelerate the shift from hospital to community services by faster development of local authority services, including help for families with mentally handicapped members living at home, residential homes for those who cannot live with their families but do not need hospital treatment, and facilities for training and occupation.'* But this will not happen unless central government gives much higher priority to the build-up of community over hospital services. Throughout the parliamentary proceedings on my Bill, repetitive emphasis was placed on its relevance to mental as well as physical handicap. Infinite care was taken (not least by my friends Jack Ashley, David

---

* Hansard, 23 June 1971, col. 307.

Weitzman and Lord Longford) to make absolutely sure that its provisions, where appropriate, would be fully available to the mentally handicapped. Our purpose was to empty the anti-hospitals of those who could live in the community by increasing family support services, such as home helps, workshops, day centres and sheltered housing. We knew that this was not only feasible and in the best interests of mentally handicapped people, but also cheaper in the long run than the so-called hospital services. In pressing for the full implementation of the Chronically Sick and Disabled Persons Act, the National Association for Mental Health and other organizations working to help the mentally handicapped now want ministers to put much more of their money where their new sentiments lie. For them to refuse to do so would be to perpetuate avoidable suffering. But for the Act to be fully activated, in the service both of the mentally and physically handicapped, the need is for an entirely new system of financing local authority services as well as for increased Exchequer support.

Ministers are also deeply implicated in the continuing scandal of high unemployment among employable disabled people. The current level of unemployment among the disabled seeking work is outrageously high. For many years, it has been four to five times as high as unemployment among the able-bodied. The legislation on the employment of the disabled is neither adequate nor fully enforced. Some of the foremost experts in this field question whether even some of the biggest employers take their legal quota of disabled employees. Many alleged fiddles are reported, such as inclusion of the names of non-disabled people in the quota. Whatever view is taken of the present system, it clearly does not prevent a wholly unacceptable level of unemployment among disabled people seeking work. Many of them crave the right to work simply to achieve or restore a sense of independence. They want the dignity of being taxpayers, not the dependence of supplementary benefits, but they are mocked by the system. What then shall be done? The legal requirement on employers to have three per cent of their employees who are registered as disabled has produced up to twelve per cent unemployment among the employable disabled. We must now, therefore, either supplement the percentage system, by the inception of new public enterprises for the employment of disabled people, or increase the legal requirement above three per cent. At the beginning of 1972, only 12,000 disabled people were employed in Remploy, local authority sheltered workshops and those of the voluntary organizations. If the legal requirement is to stay unchanged, this number must be substantially increased. We must also ensure that the law, whatever it says, is fully enforced. In turn, that will mean improving access and egress for disabled people at more and more places of work. There are many disabled people who have been offered jobs only to find it impossible to take them because of difficulties of access and egress or the lack of suitable facilities inside the place of work. If investment in adaptations is what is required, it is for Ministers to encourage this by financial incentives. The new chairmobile, inspired by Lord Snowdon and financed by the *Sunday Mirror*, is an example of what can be done to improve the indoor mobility of severely disabled people. If such aids make it easier for any disabled person to find and retain employment, it is in the taxpayer's interest that they should be provided. Here again, there is no *saving* in failing to spend the amount of public money necessary to increase the independence of disabled people.

Improving the employment opportunities of the disabled also means improving their outdoor mobility. There are many disabled people who cannot fulfil their ambition to seek work because they are still denied adequate means of mobility outside the home. Even many of the severely disabled people who receive help with their mobility are given vehicles which are totally unsuited to their needs. It is not just that the three-wheeler, with its one seat, disrupts the family lives of disabled people. This vehicle is of little real use to the disabled person who needs to be helped in and out of a car. Yet my researches show that it costs no more to provide a disabled person with a four-wheeled vehicle than with the three-wheeler. Motor manufacturers confirm that they could supply a four-wheeled vehicle with the necessary

adaptations that would be no more expensive, per car, than
the Ministry's three-wheeler. Why then are Ministers
apparently so wrong-headed? The reason is that, if they were
to provide suitable vehicles for the physically handicapped,
there would be a sharp increase in the number of entitled
applicants. It is rather like offering distasteful sweets, not
because they are cheaper, but because fewer people will want
them. The result is that people who could work and become
taxpayers, if only they were given proper help with mobility,
are made to regard themselves as unemployable. Instead
of working, they deteriorate in enforced idleness; instead
of living, they exist. Minor improvements in the Ministry's
vehicle service are welcome. But as I have argued in the
Commons, they are no substitute for a realization by
Ministers that investment in people, disabled people no
less than fit and strong and fortunate people, is the best of
all investments.

In the Act's provisions to help deaf-blind, dyslexic and
autistic children, as well as children suffering from other
forms of early childhood psychosis, we have the means
rapidly to improve the educational standards of these
children. This was another of the deeply sensitive problems
to which many of my parliamentary colleagues addressed
themselves when my Bill was being drafted. Jack Ashley had
made a very close study of the treatment of the three categories of severely disabled children covered by Sections
(25)-(27) of the Act. His was a superb contribution to our
work in drafting these provisions. But there is still a grave
inadequacy in public provision for the special educational
needs of these three categories of children. Voluntary
organizations have striven heroically to cope with this inadequacy. The National Society for Autistic Children alone
set out to raise £100,000 because of the total lack, in many
localities, of educational facilities for children suffering from
autism. Under Sections (25)-(27) of the Act, there is now
much more that the Secretary of State for Education and
Science can do to stimulate local education authorities to
satisfy the special needs of deaf-blind, dyslexic and autistic
children. The three sections emphasize the compellingly

urgent need for *public* provision to meet the needs of these children. Their intention is to ensure that society as a whole discharges the duty to cater for its children in special need. Yet the voluntary societies have put much more drive into publicising the new provisions than the statutory bodies have shown in implementing them. Local initiatives can be extremely important in translating Sections (25)-(27) into full public provision. It is for all of us, in our localities, to see to it that these sections of the Act are not invalidated by local inaction. Local initiatives are not, however, enough by themselves. Ministers must also play their part. If necessary, they should provide new and special incentives for the local education authorities to act. After all, there was no party difference about the urgency of the case for full public provision when my Bill was debated by Parliament. There are cases of unsatisfied need, especially among autistic children, where urgency has never been more urgent. For Ministers to delay in helping these cases is to make higher public expenditure in the future an unavoidable certainty.

The financial problems of most disabled people have been frequently acknowledged throughout this book. They are problems that cannot be solved overnight. But it is essential that every improvement we make is conceived as part of a long-term plan for the rehabilitation of disabled people and for their full integration into the community. The constant attendance allowance first proposed by Richard Crossman was brought into force by his successor as Secretary of State for the Social Services. The rigidity of the definition of eligibility has inevitably caused keen disappointment among tens of thousands of very hard-pressed but unsuccessful applicants. Even though if the definition is being extended to cover a much wider category of disabled people, the allowance must be regarded only as a modest first step toward plans for a national disability income. Such an income might be one payable to all who are severely disabled, physically or mentally, whatever the cause of their disabilities and regardless of when they occurred. This would end the injustice of regarding disabled housewives and many disabled children as if they were non-persons. Income

would be linked to need, instead of being related, as it is
now, to the *cause* of disablement. The financial effects of
disability are twofold. First, there is loss of earning capacity;
and secondly, the extra living costs of being disabled.
A national disability income would need to take both effects
into account. To encourage rehabilitation, payment of
part of the income might be continued to disabled people
who achieve, or regain a limited capacity for work. By
preference, this would be assessed, not by reference to the
disabled person's loss of faculty, but to his residual earning
ability compared with that of the average able-bodied person.
The cost of the scheme would be offset, first, by a saving in
means-tested supplementary benefits; secondly, by fewer
disabled people needing long-stay institutional care and
fewer of their children the care of local authorities; and
thirdly, by increased use of the working capacity of disabled
people. The viability of such a scheme merits urgent study by
central government. Ministers must also unequivocally
accept that it is *net* cost, not apparent cost, that should now
inform the making of policy on disablement income. For it
is the absence of any real attempt to measure net cost that
has produced policies that are neither cheap nor efficient nor
humane.

One of the central purposes of my Bill was to challenge
what Sir William Oastler called that ' . . . serene satisfaction
with the *status quo*'. The new Act has been most warmly
welcomed by all the voluntary organizations working among
handicapped people. But there is still much to do if we are to
turn precept and law into administrative practice and full
social provision. The problem still facing us is a vast one
requiring every organization, statutory and voluntary alike,
to discuss their priorities. We need a blueprint which provides
for resources to be used as humanely and effectively as
possible and to the maximum efficiency of the handicapped.
None of the very wide fellowship who helped to make and
enact my Bill ever doubted the size and gravity of the task
we confronted. Yet we hoped, by working together, that we
could change the *status quo* for Britain's disabled and end the
'serene satisfaction' by which they were oppressed. My own

approach to disablement was expressed in the speech with which I presented my Bill for Second Reading in the House of Commons. It is that we must seek a society in which there is genuine respect for the handicapped; where understanding is unostentatious and sincere; where if years cannot be added to the lives of the very sick, at least life can be added to their years; where needs come before means; where the mobility of disabled people is restricted only by the bounds of technical progress and discovery; where the handicapped have a fundamental right to participate in industry and society according to ability; where socially preventable distress is unknown; and where no man has cause to feel ill-at-ease because of his disability.

Appendix

~~~~~~

Chronically Sick and Disabled Persons Act 1970

Chronically Sick and Disabled Persons Act 1970

CHAPTER 44

ARRANGEMENT OF SECTIONS

ELIZABETH II

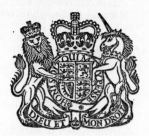

1970 CHAPTER 44

An Act to make further provision with respect to the welfare of chronically sick and disabled persons; and for connected purposes.　　　　[29th May 1970]

BE IT ENACTED by the Queen's most Excellent Majesty, by and with the advice and consent of the Lords Spiritual and Temporal, and Commons, in this present Parliament assembled, and by the authority of the same, as follows:—

Welfare and housing

1.—(1) It shall be the duty of every local authority having functions under section 29 of the National Assistance Act 1948 to inform themselves of the number of persons to whom that section applies within their area and of the need for the making by the authority of arrangements under that section for such persons. *Information as to need for and existence of welfare services.* *1948 c. 29.*

(2) Every such local authority—

　(*a*) shall cause to be published from time to time at such times and in such manner as they consider appropriate general information as to the services provided under arrangements made by the authority under the said section 29 which are for the time being available in their area; and

　(*b*) shall ensure that any such person as aforesaid who uses any of those services is informed of any other of those services which in the opinion of the authority is relevant to his needs.

(3) This section shall come into operation on such date as the Secretary of State may by order made by statutory instrument appoint.

A 2

Provision
of welfare
services.
1948 c. 29.

2.—(1) Where a local authority having functions under section 29 of the National Assistance Act 1948 are satisfied in the case of any person to whom that section applies who is ordinarily resident in their area that it is necessary in order to meet the needs of that person for that authority to make arrangements for all or any of the following matters, namely—

(*a*) the provision of practical assistance for that person in his home;

(*b*) the provision for that person of, or assistance to that person in obtaining, wireless, television, library or similar recreational facilities;

(*c*) the provision for that person of lectures, games, outings or other recreational facilities outside his home or assistance to that person in taking advantage of educational facilities available to him;

(*d*) the provision for that person of facilities for, or assistance in, travelling to and from his home for the purpose of participating in any services provided under arrangements made by the authority under the said section 29 or, with the approval of the authority, in any services provided otherwise than as aforesaid which are similar to services which could be provided under such arrangements;

(*e*) the provision of assistance for that person in arranging for the carrying out of any works of adaptation in his home or the provision of any additional facilities designed to secure his greater safety, comfort or convenience;

(*f*) facilitating the taking of holidays by that person, whether at holiday homes or otherwise and whether provided under arrangements made by the authority or otherwise;

(*g*) the provision of meals for that person whether in his home or elsewhere;

(*h*) the provision for that person of, or assistance to that person in obtaining, a telephone and any special equipment necessary to enable him to use a telephone,

then, notwithstanding anything in any scheme made by the authority under the said section 29, but subject to the provisions of section 35(2) of that Act (which requires local authorities to exercise their functions under Part III of that Act under the general guidance of the Secretary of State and in accordance with the provisions of any regulations made for the purpose), it shall be the duty of that authority to make those arrangements in exercise of their functions under the said section 29.

(2) Without prejudice to the said section 35(2), subsection (3) of the said section 29 (which requires any arrangements made by

a local authority under that section to be carried into effect in accordance with a scheme made thereunder) shall not apply—

(a) to any arrangements made in pursuance of subsection (1) of this section; or

(b) in the case of a local authority who have made such a scheme, to any arrangements made by virtue of subsection (1) of the said section 29 in addition to those required or authorised by the scheme which are so made with the approval of the Secretary of State.

3.—(1) Every local authority for the purposes of Part V of the Housing Act 1957 in discharging their duty under section 91 of that Act to consider housing conditions in their district and the needs of the district with respect to the provision of further housing accommodation shall have regard to the special needs of chronically sick or disabled persons; and any proposals prepared and submitted to the Minister by the authority under that section for the provision of new houses shall distinguish any houses which the authority propose to provide which make special provision for the needs of such persons. *Duties of housing authorities. 1957 c. 56.*

(2) In the application of this section to Scotland for the words "Part V of the Housing Act 1957", "91" and "Minister" there shall be substituted respectively the words "Part VII of the Housing (Scotland) Act 1966", "137" and "Secretary of State". *1966 c. 49.*

Premises open to public

4.—(1) Any person undertaking the provision of any building or premises to which the public are to be admitted, whether on payment or otherwise, shall, in the means of access both to and within the building or premises, and in the parking facilities and sanitary conveniences to be available (if any), make provision, in so far as it is in the circumstances both practicable and reasonable, for the needs of members of the public visiting the building or premises who are disabled. *Access to, and facilities at, premises open to the public.*

(2) This section shall not apply to any building or premises intended for purposes mentioned in subsection (2) of section 8 of this Act.

5.—(1) Where any local authority undertake the provision of a public sanitary convenience, it shall be the duty of the authority, in doing so, to make provision, in so far as it is in the circumstances both practicable and reasonable, for the needs of disabled persons. *Provision of public sanitary conveniences.*

(2) Any local authority which in any public sanitary convenience provided by them make or have made provision for the needs of disabled persons shall take such steps as may be reasonable, by sign-posts or similar notices, to indicate the whereabouts of the convenience.

1933 c. 51.
1947 c. 43.

(3) In this section "local authority" means a local authority within the meaning of the Local Government Act 1933 or the Local Government (Scotland) Act 1947 and any joint board or joint committee of which all the constituent authorities are local authorities within the meaning of either of those Acts.

Provision of sanitary conveniences at certain premises open to the public.
1936 c. 49.

6.—(1) Any person upon whom a notice is served with respect to any premises under section 89 of the Public Health Act 1936 (which empowers local authorities by notice to make requirements as to the provision and maintenance of sanitary conveniences for the use of persons frequenting certain premises used for the accommodation, refreshment or entertainment of members of the public) shall in complying with that notice make provision, in so far as it is in the circumstances both practicable and reasonable, for the needs of persons frequenting those premises who are disabled.

1959 c. 24.

(2) The owner of a building, who has been ordered under section 11(4) of the Building (Scotland) Act 1959 to make the building conform to a provision of building standards regulations made under section 3 of that Act requiring the provision of suitable and sufficient sanitary conveniences therein, shall in complying with that order make provision, in so far as it is in the circumstances both practicable and reasonable, for the needs of persons frequenting that building who are disabled.

Signs at buildings complying with ss. 4–6.

7.—(1) Where any provision required by or under section 4, 5 or 6 of this Act is made at a building in compliance with that section, a notice or sign indicating that provision is made for the disabled shall be displayed outside the building or so as to be visible from outside it.

(2) This section applies to a sanitary convenience provided elsewhere than in a building, and not itself being a building, as it applies to a building.

University and school buildings

Access to, and facilities at, university and school buildings.

8.—(1) Any person undertaking the provision of a building intended for purposes mentioned in subsection (2) below shall, in the means of access both to and within the building, and in the parking facilities and sanitary conveniences to be available (if any), make provision, in so far as it is in the circumstances both practicable and reasonable, for the needs of persons using the building who are disabled.

(2) The purposes referred to in subsection (1) above are the purposes of any of the following:—

    (a) universities, university colleges and colleges, schools and halls of universities;

(*b*) schools within the meaning of the Education Act 1944, 1944 c. 31.
teacher training colleges maintained by local education
authorities in England or Wales and other institutions
providing further education pursuant to a scheme under
section 42 of that Act;

(*c*) educational establishments within the meaning of the
Education (Scotland) Act 1962. · 1962 c. 37.

Advisory committees, etc.

9.—(1) The Secretary of State shall ensure that the central Central
advisory committee constituted under section 3 of the War advisory
Pensions Act 1921 includes the chairmen of not less than twelve committee
of the committees established by schemes under section 1 of that pensions.
Act and includes at least one war disabled pensioner, and shall 1921 c. 49.
cause that central advisory committee to be convened at least
once in every year.

(2) This section extends to Northern Ireland.

10. In the appointment of persons to be members of the Central Housing
Housing Advisory Committee set up under section 143 of the Advisory
Housing Act 1957 or of the Scottish Housing Advisory Committee Committees.
set up under section 167 of the Housing (Scotland) Act 1966, 1957 c. 56.
regard shall be had to the desirability of that Committee's 1966 c. 49.
including one or more persons with knowledge of the problems
involved in housing the chronically sick and disabled and to the
person or persons with that knowledge being or including a
chronically sick or disabled person or persons.

11. The National Insurance Advisory Committee shall include National
at least one person with experience of work among and of the Insurance
needs of the chronically sick and disabled and in selecting any Advisory
such person regard shall be had to the desirability of having a Committee.
chronically sick or disabled person.

12. The Industrial Injuries Advisory Council shall include at Industrial
least one person with experience of work among and of the Injuries
needs of the chronically sick and disabled and in selecting any Advisory
such person regard shall be had to the desirability of having a Council.
chronically sick or disabled person.

13.—(1) Without prejudice to any other arrangements that Youth·
may be made by the Secretary of State, the Central Youth employment
Employment Executive shall include at least one person with service.
special responsibility for the employment of young disabled
persons.

(2) In the appointment of persons to be members of any of
the bodies constituted in pursuance of section 8(1) of the Employment and Training Act 1948 (that is to say, the National Youth 1948 c. 46.

Employment Council and the Advisory Committees on Youth Employment for Scotland and Wales respectively) regard shall be had to the desirability of the body in question including one or more persons with experience of work among, and the special needs of, young disabled persons and to the person or persons with that experience being or including a disabled person or persons.

Miscellaneous advisory committees.

14.—(1) In the appointment of persons to be members of any of the following advisory committees or councils, that is to say, the Transport Users' Consultative Committees, the Gas Consultative Councils, the Electricity Consultative Councils, the Post Office Users' Councils and the Domestic Coal Consumers' Council; regard shall be had to the desirability of the committee or council in question including one or more persons with experience of work among, and the special needs of, disabled persons and to the person or persons with that experience being or including a disabled person or persons.

(2) In this section the reference to the Post Office Users' Councils is a reference to the Councils established under section 14 of the Post Office Act 1969, and in relation to those Councils this section shall extend to Northern Ireland.

1969 c. 48.

Co-option of chronically sick or disabled persons to local authority committees.
1933 c. 51.
1947 c. 43.

15. Where a local authority within the meaning of the Local Government Act 1933 or the Local Government (Scotland) Act 1947 appoint a committee of the authority under any enactment, and the members of the committee include or may include persons who are not members of the authority, then in considering the appointment to the committee of such persons regard shall be had, if the committee is concerned with matters in which the chronically sick or disabled have special needs, to the desirability of appointing to the committee persons with experience of work among and of the needs of the chronically sick and disabled, and to the person or persons with that experience being or including a chronically sick or disabled person or persons.

Duties of national advisory council under Disabled Persons (Employment) Act 1944.
1944 c. 10.

16. The duties of the national advisory council established under section 17(1)(*a*) of the Disabled Persons (Employment) Act 1944 shall include in particular the duty of giving to the Secretary of State such advice as appears to the council to be necessary on the training of persons concerned with—

    (*a*) placing disabled persons in employment; or

    (*b*) training disabled persons for employment.

Provisions with respect to persons under 65

17.—(1) Every Board constituted under section 11 of the National Health Service Act 1946 (that is to say, every Regional Hospital Board and every Board of Governors of a teaching hospital) and every Regional Hospital Board constituted under section 11 of the National Health Service (Scotland) Act 1947 shall use their best endeavours to secure that, so far as practicable, in any hospital for which they are responsible a person who is suffering from a condition of chronic illness or disability and who— Separation of younger from older patients.
1946 c. 81.
1947 c. 27.

    (*a*) is in the hospital for the purpose of long-term care for that condition; or

    (*b*) normally resides elsewhere but is being cared for in the hospital because—

        (i) that condition is such as to preclude him from residing elsewhere without the assistance of some other person; and

        (ii) such assistance is for the time being not available,

is not cared for in the hospital as an in-patient in any part of the hospital which is normally used wholly or mainly for the care of elderly persons, unless he is himself an elderly person.

  (2) Each such Board as aforesaid shall provide the Secretary of State in such form and at such times as he may direct with such information as he may from time to time require as to any persons to whom subsection (1) of this section applied who, not being elderly persons, have been cared for in any hospital for which that Board are responsible in such a part of the hospital as is mentioned in that subsection; and the Secretary of State shall in each year lay before each House of Parliament such statement in such form as he considers appropriate of the information obtained by him under this subsection.

  (3) In this section " elderly person " means a person who is aged sixty-five or more or is suffering from the effects of premature ageing.

18.—(1) The Secretary of State shall take steps to obtain from local authorities having functions under Part III of the National Assistance Act 1948 information as to the number of persons under the age of 65 appearing to the local authority in question to be persons to whom section 29 of that Act applies for whom residential accommodation is from time to time provided under section 21(1)(*a*) or 26(1)(*a*) of that Act at any premises in a part of those premises in which such accommodation is so provided for persons over that age. Information as to accommodation of younger persons under Part III of National Assistance Act 1948.
1948 c. 29.

1968 c. 49.

1960 c. 61.

(2) The Secretary of State shall take steps to obtain from local authorities having functions under the Social Work (Scotland) Act 1968 information as to the number of persons under the age of 65 who suffer from illness or mental disorder within the meaning of section 6 of the Mental Health (Scotland) Act 1960 or are substantially handicapped by any deformity or disability and for whom residential accommodation is from time to time provided under section 59 of the said Act of 1968 at any premises in a part of those premises in which such accommodation is so provided for persons over that age.

(3) Every local authority referred to in this section shall provide the Secretary of State in such form and at such times as he may direct with such information as he may from time to time require for the purpose of this section; and the Secretary of State shall in each year lay before each House of Parliament such statement in such form as he considers appropriate of the information obtained by him under this section.

Provision of information relating to chiropody services.

1968 c. 46.

1947 c. 27.

19. Every local health authority empowered to provide chiropody services under section 12 of the Health Services and Public Health Act 1968, or under section 27 of the National Health Service (Scotland) Act 1947, shall provide the Secretary of State in such form and at such times as he may direct with information as to the extent to which those services are available and used for the benefit of disabled persons under the age of sixty-five.

Miscellaneous provisions

Use of invalid carriages on highways.

20.—(1) In the case of a vehicle which is an invalid carriage complying with the prescribed requirements and which is being used in accordance with the prescribed conditions—

    (*a*) no statutory provision prohibiting or restricting the use of footways shall prohibit or restrict the use of that vehicle on a footway;

1960 c. 16.
1962 c. 59.
1967 c. 76.
1967 c. 30.

    (*b*) if the vehicle is mechanically propelled, it shall be treated for the purposes of the Road Traffic Act 1960, the Road Traffic Act 1962, the Road Traffic Regulation Act 1967 and Part I of the Road Safety Act 1967 as not being a motor vehicle; and

1957 c. 51.

    (*c*) whether or not the vehicle is mechanically propelled, it shall be exempted from the requirements of the Road Transport Lighting Act 1957.

(2) In this section—

1959 c. 25.

    " footway " means a way which is a footway, footpath or bridleway within the meaning of the Highways Act 1959;

and in its application to Scotland means a way over
which the public has a right of passage on foot only or a
bridleway within the meaning of section 47 of the
Countryside (Scotland) Act 1967;   1967 c. 86.

"invalid carriage" means a vehicle, whether mechanically
propelled or not, constructed or adapted for use for the
carriage of one person, being a person suffering from
some physical defect or disability;

"prescribed" means prescribed by regulations made by the
Minister of Transport;

"statutory provision" means a provision contained in, or
having effect under, any enactment.

(3) Any regulations made under this section shall be made by
statutory instrument, may make different provision for different
circumstances and shall be subject to annulment in pursuance of
a resolution of either House of Parliament.

21.—(1) There shall be a badge of a prescribed form to be Badges for
issued by local authorities for motor vehicles driven by, or used display
for the carriage of, disabled persons; and— on motor
                                                        vehicles used
(a) subject to the provisions of this section, the badge so by disabled
issued for any vehicle or vehicles may be displayed on persons.
it or on any of them either inside or outside the area
of the issuing authority; and

(b) any power under section 84C of the Road Traffic Regula- 1967 c. 76.
tion Act 1967 (which was inserted by the Transport 1968 c. 73.
Act 1968) to make regulations requiring that orders
under the Act shall include exemptions shall be taken
to extend to requiring that an exemption given with
reference to badges issued by one authority shall be
given also with reference to badges issued by other
authorities.

(2) A badge may be issued to a disabled person of any prescribed description resident in the area of the issuing authority
for one or more vehicles which he drives and, if so issued, may
be displayed on it or any of them at times when he is the driver.

(3) In such cases as may be prescribed, a badge may be issued
to a disabled person of any prescribed description so resident
for one or more vehicles used by him as a passenger and, if so
issued, may be displayed on it or any of them at times when the
vehicle is being used to carry him.

A badge may be issued to the same person both under this
subsection and under subsection (2) above.

(4) A badge may be issued to an institution concerned with
the care of the disabled for any motor vehicle or, as the case

may be, for each motor vehicle kept in the area of the issuing authority and used by or on behalf of the institution to carry disabled persons of any prescribed description; and any badge so issued may be displayed on the vehicle for which it is issued at times when the vehicle is being so used.

(5) A local authority shall maintain a register showing the holders of badges issued by the authority under this section, and the vehicle or vehicles for which each of the badges is held; and in the case of badges issued to disabled persons the register shall show whether they were, for any motor vehicle, issued under subsection (2) or under subsection (3) or both.

(6) A badge issued under this section shall remain the property of the issuing authority, shall be issued for such period as may be prescribed, and shall be returned to the issuing authority in such circumstances as may be prescribed.

(7) Anything which is under this section to be prescribed shall be prescribed by regulations made by the Minister of Transport and Secretary of State by statutory instrument, which shall be subject to annulment in pursuance of a resolution of either House of Parliament; and regulations so made may make provision—

(*a*) as to the cases in which authorities may refuse to issue badges, and as to the fee (if any) which an authority may charge for the issue or re-issue of a badge; and

1948 c. 29.

(*b*) as to the continuing validity or effect of badges issued before the coming into force of this section in pursuance of any scheme having effect under section 29 of the National Assistance Act 1948 or any similar scheme having effect in Scotland; and

1967 c. 76.

(*c*) as to any transitional matters, and in particular the application to badges issued under this section of orders made before it comes into force and operating with reference to any such badges as are referred to in paragraph (*b*) above (being orders made, or having effect as if made, under the Road Traffic Regulation Act 1967).

(8) The local authorities for purposes of this section shall be the common council of the City of London, the council of a county or county borough in England or Wales or of a London borough and the council of a county or large burgh in Scotland; and in this section " motor vehicle " has the same meaning as in the Road Traffic Regulation Act 1967.

(9) This section shall come into operation on such date as the Minister of Transport and Secretary of State may by order made by statutory instrument appoint.

22. The Secretary of State shall as respects each year lay before Parliament a report on the progress made during that year in research and development work carried out by or on behalf of any Minister of the Crown in relation to equipment that might increase the range of activities and independence or well-being of disabled persons, and in particular such equipment that might improve the indoor and outdoor mobility of such persons.

Annual report on research and development work.

23.—(1) The Pensions Appeal Tribunals Act 1943 shall have effect with the amendments specified in the subsequent provisions of this section.

War pensions appeals.

1943 c. 39.

(2) In section 5—

> (*a*) so much of subsection (1) as prevents the making of an appeal from an interim assessment of the degree of a disablement before the expiration of two years from the first notification of the making of an interim assessment (that is to say, the words from " if " to " subsection " where first occurring, and the words " in force at the expiration of the said period of two years ") is hereby repealed except in relation to a claim in the case of which the said first notification was given before the commencement of this Act;

> (*b*) in the second paragraph of subsection (1) (which defines " interim assessment " for the purposes of that subsection), for the words " this subsection " there shall be substituted the words " this section ";

> (*c*) in subsection (2) (which provides for an appeal to a tribunal from a Ministerial decision or assessment purporting to be a final settlement of a claim) at the end there shall be added the words " and if the Tribunal so set aside the Minister's decision or assessment they may, if they think fit, make such interim assessment of the degree or nature of the disablement, to be in force until such date not later than two years after the making of the Tribunal's assessment, as they think proper ";

> (*d*) subsection (3) (which makes provision as to the coming into operation of section 5) is hereby repealed.

(3) In section 6, after subsection (2) there shall be inserted the following subsection—

> " (2A) Where, in the case of such a claim as is referred to in section 1, 2, 3 or 4 of this Act—

>> (*a*) an appeal has been made under that section to the Tribunal and that appeal has been decided (whether with or without an appeal under subsection (2) of this section from the Tribunal's decision); but

(*b*) subsequently, on an application for the purpose made (in like manner as an application for leave to appeal under the said subsection (2)) jointly by the appellant and the Minister, it appears to the appropriate authority (that is to say, the person to whom under rules made under the Schedule to this Act any application for directions on any matter arising in connection with the appeal to the Tribunal fell to be made) to be proper so to do—

(i) by reason of the availability of additional evidence; or

(ii) (except where an appeal from the Tribunal's decision has been made under the said subsection (2)), on the ground of the Tribunal's decision being erroneous in point of law,

the appropriate authority may, if he thinks fit, direct that the decision on the appeal to the Tribunal be treated as set aside and the appeal from the Minister's decision be heard again by the Tribunal ".

(4) In subsection (3) of section 6 (under which, subject to subsection (2) of that section, a tribunal's decision is final and conclusive) for the words " subject to the last foregoing sub-section " there shall be substituted the words " subject to sub-sections (2) and (2A) of this section ".

S.I. 1968/1699.

(5) In consequence of the Secretary of State for Social Services Order 1968, in section 12(1), for the definition of " the Minister " there shall be substituted the following:—

". ' the Minister '. means the Secretary of State for Social Services ".

(6) This section extends to Northern Ireland.

Institute of hearing research.

24. The Secretary of State shall collate and present evidence to the Medical Research Council on the need for an institute for hearing research, such institute to have the general function of co-ordinating and promoting research on hearing and assistance to the deaf and hard of hearing.

Special educational treatment for the deaf-blind.

25.—(1) It shall be the duty of every local education authority to provide the Secretary of State at such times as he may direct with information on the provision made by that local education authority of special educational facilities for children who suffer the dual handicap of blindness and deafness.

(2) The arrangements made by a local education authority for the special educational treatment of the deaf-blind shall, so far as is practicable, provide for the giving of such education in any school maintained or assisted by the local education authority.

(3) In the application of this section to Scotland for any reference to a local education authority there shall be substituted a reference to an education authority within the meaning of section 145 of the Education (Scotland) Act 1962.

1962 c. 47.

26.—(1) It shall be the duty of every local education authority to provide the Secretary of State at such times as he may direct with information on the provision made by that local education authority of special educational facilities for children who suffer from autism or other forms of early childhood psychosis.

Special educational treatment for children suffering from autism, &c.

(2) The arrangements made by a local education authority for the special educational treatment of children suffering from autism and other forms of early childhood psychosis shall, so far as is practicable, provide for the giving of such education in any school maintained or assisted by the local education authority.

(3) In the application of this section to Scotland for any reference to a local education authority there shall be substituted a reference to an education authority within the meaning of section 145 of the Education (Scotland) Act 1962.

27.—(1) It shall be the duty of every local education authority to provide the Secretary of State at such times as he may direct with information on the provision made by that local education authority of special educational facilities for children who suffer from acute dyslexia.

Special educational treatment for children suffering from acute dyslexia.

(2) The arrangements made by a local education authority for the special educational treatment of children suffering from acute dyslexia shall, so far as is practicable, provide for the giving of such education in any school maintained or assisted by the local education authority.

(3) In the application of this section to Scotland for any reference to a local education authority there shall be substituted a reference to an education authority within the meaning of section 145 of the Education (Scotland) Act 1962.

28. Where it appears to the Secretary of State to be necessary or expedient to do so for the proper operation of any provision of this Act, he may by regulations made by statutory instrument, which shall be subject to annulment in pursuance of a resolution of either House of Parliament, make provision as to the interpretation for the purposes of that provision of any of the following expressions appearing therein, that is to say, " chronically sick ", " chronic illness ", " disabled " and " disability ".

Power to define certain expressions.

29.—(1) This Act may be cited as the Chronically Sick and Disabled Persons Act 1970.

Short title, extent and commencement.

(2) Sections 1 and 2 of this Act do not extend to Scotland.

(3) Save as otherwise expressly provided by sections 9, 14 and 23, this Act does not extend to Northern Ireland.

(4) This Act shall come into force as follows:—

    (*a*) sections 1 and 21 shall come into force on the day appointed thereunder;

    (*b*) sections 4, 5, 6, 7 and 8 shall come into force at the expiration of six months beginning with the date this Act is passed;

    (*c*) the remainder shall come into force at the expiration of three months beginning with that date.

PRINTED IN ENGLAND BY C. H. BAYLIS, C.B.

Controller of Her Majesty's Stationery Office and Queen's Printer of Acts of Parliament

Fourth Impression June 1971

LONDON: PUBLISHED BY HER MAJESTY'S STATIONERY OFFICE

12½p net

Index